Bilingual Advantages

Linguistic Insights

Studies in Language and Communication

Edited by Maurizio Gotti,
University of Bergamo

Volume 213

PETER LANG
Bern · Berlin · Bruxelles · Frankfurt am Main · New York · Oxford · Wien

Zhilong Xie

Bilingual Advantages

Contributions of Different Bilingual Experiences
to Cognitive Control Differences
Among Young-adult Bilinguals

PETER LANG
Bern · Berlin · Bruxelles · Frankfurt am Main · New York · Oxford · Wien

Bibliographic information published by die Deutsche Nationalbibliothek
Die Deutsche Nationalbibliothek lists this publication in the Deutsche Nationalbibliografie; detailed bibliographic data is available on the Internet at ‹http://dnb.d-nb.de›.

British Library Cataloguing-in-Publication Data: A catalogue record for this book is available from The British Library, Great Britain.

Library of Congress Control Number: 2016941922

Dissertation
Presented in Partial Fulfillment of the Requirements for the Degree of Doctor of Philosophy in Psycholinguistics
Supervisor: Dong, Yanping; Guangdong University of Foreign Studies

The research is supported by National Social Science Foundation of China (15AYY002).

ISSN 1424-8689 pb. ISSN 2235-6371 eBook
ISBN 978-3-0343-2081-8 pb. ISBN 978-3-0351-0938-2 eBook

This publication has been peer reviewed.

Hochfeldstrasse 32, CH-3012 Bern, Switzerland
info@peterlang.com, www.peterlang.com

Acknowledgements

Without the encouragement and help from many people, the completion of this study would never have been possible.

I am, in particular, deeply indebted to my PhD supervisor, Professor Yanping Dong, who has always been an inspiration and a star to me. Without her insightful guidance and strict discipline, this volume could never have reached the present form.

I was also greatly indebted to Professor Jianda Liu for his generous help and encouragement in my life and study.

I owe much gratitude to our team under the guidance of Professor Yanping Dong. Without their help and critical suggestions in our seminars, I could have been stuck in many of the hard situations.

I owe a great debt of gratitude to Professor Yongshou Huo, Professor Xudong Wu, and Professor Chen Zhao for their invaluable suggestions and relevant PhD course instructions during the three years of my study in GDUFS.

I am thankful particularly to Mr. Khashi Shahbzi for his generous help in language editing.

I also owe a great debt of gratitude to Professor Zhenhui Rao, Professor Yongzhong Li, Professor Chunyan Liu, and Professor Yuying Li from Foreign Languages College in Jiangxi Normal University for their support and help to my research by generously providing me with experiment facilities whenever I was in need.

I am especially grateful to Professor Fagen Li, and Professor Yuewu Lin, for their assistance and help to me and my family. Thanks are also extended to all the students from Guangdong University of Foreign Studies and to all the students from Jiangxi Normal University, who participated in the experiments of this research.

My gratitude also goes to my wife – Xiaoxia He, my daughter – Jiming Xie, my parents, and my parents-in-law for their love and support.

Contents

Chapter 1: Bilingual Experience and Cognitive Control

More and more people in this world today are speaking two (or more) languages. Speaking two languages makes language processing very complicated. Moreover, managing two languages places huge demands on the cognitive system and therefore may affect many aspects of cognitive development. Accumulating evidence has shown that bilingual experience has a systematic and significant impact on cognitive control. What remains unresolved is how a specific bilingual experience contributes to changes of cognitive control. The current research intends to shed light on this issue.

1.1 Introduction

Some early studies (e.g., Saer, 1923; Smith, 1923) report that learning two languages is detrimental to bilingual learners' intelligence. In later years, it was reported that the vocabulary size of monolinguals is larger than that of bilinguals in that language (Pearson, Fernandez, & Oller, 1993). This result is also supported by a more recent study (Bialystok, Luk, Peets, & Yang, 2010), which finds that the mean standard of monolinguals is reliably higher than that of compared bilinguals. Therefore, it is reasonable to assume that learning two languages may cause some disadvantages to bilinguals.

However, more and more studies have shown that for bilinguals learning two languages, this learning has a significant and positive impact on their cognitive functioning. A study by Peal and Lambert (1962) initiated a significant trend of research on bilingual advantage. They found that bilinguals have an advantage on tests requiring symbol manipulation and reorganization. They suggest that having to switch between the two languages might be the reason that causes the enhanced mental flexibility, superiority in concept formation, and diversified mental abilities (Peal & Lambert, 1962).

More recently, the effect of bilingualism on cognitive control has been an area of great interest. Much research suggests that bilinguals have advantage over their monolingual counterparts when they perform cognitive control tasks (Bialystok, 2011; Bialystok, Craik, Klein, & Viswanathan, 2004; Bialystok, Craik, Green, & Gollan, 2009; Bialystok, Craik, & Ryan, 2006). This cognitive control advantage has been detected among child bilinguals relative to their monolingual peers (e.g., Bialystok, Barac, Blaye, & Poulin-Dubois, 2010) and among older adult bilinguals who showed delayed cognitive decline compared with their monolingual counterparts (e.g., Bialystok, Craik, & Freedman, 2007). In fact, some studies have also shown that young-adult bilinguals have cognitive control advantage relative to their counterpart monolinguals, at least in some cognitive control tasks (Bialystok, 2009; Costa, Hernandez, Costa-Faidella, & Sebastian-Galles, 2009; Prior & Gollan, 2011; Prior & Macwhinney, 2010), although a few studies have failed to capture this advantage, particularly in behavioral measures under low cognitive demand (Bialystok, Craik, & Ryan, 2006; Costa et al., 2009; Luk, Anderson, Craik, Grady, & Bialystok, 2010).

Besides behavioral results, ERPs (Event related potentials) studies show that there is a language control mechanism required to regulate and control the use of different languages and to prevent interference between them. In a recent study, an inhibitory effect (N200) was detected in on-line bilingual processing (Moreno, Rodrıguez-Fornells, & Laine, 2008). Moreover, in functional and structural neuroimaging studies (fMRI) (e.g., Abutalebi et al., 2012; Hervais-Adelman, Moser-Mercer, Michel, & Golestani, 2014) it is demonstrated that a structure tightly bound to domain-general cognitive control functions (e.g., dorsal anterior cingulate cortex ACC, the caudate nucleus), is a common locus for language control and resolving nonverbal conflict. Because of the need to switch between two alternate languages and because of the need to inhibit one over the other in order to use the target language, bilinguals use this common locus more frequently and more efficiently than monolinguals, so this advantage in language control very likely transfers to resolving nonlinguistic cognitive conflicts in domain-general cognitive control tasks, leading to bilingual advantage.

1.2 Definition of Terms

There are two general terms requiring definition for the convenience of the following discussions. More detailed descriptions and discussions of the relevant terms will be presented in the literature review section.

The first general term is *bilingualism*. Bilingualism may have different definitions in different academic fields. "Bilingualism" should be understood to include knowledge of any number of languages beyond one (Valian, 2014). For the current perspective, bilingualism refers generally to the state of speaking/learning two languages (Bialystok et al., 2009). There are two distinct categories of bilingualism. The first is simultaneous bilingualism in which people take one language as the official language and at the same time take another language as their daily language in life. In this category, the learning of two languages often takes place simultaneously at early childhood, and bilinguals in this case are often balanced bilingual speakers. The second type of bilingualism is sequential bilingualism in which people learn a second or foreign language in a late age after the acquisition of their mother tongue. Learning two languages takes place sequentially, and in this case bilinguals are often unbalanced bilingual speakers.

The second general term is *cognitive control,* which is also referred to as *executive control* or *executive functions* or *executive processing* in the field. Currently, it refers to the ability to control the processes that allow information processing or behavior to change flexibly according to different goals. Cognitive control processes include a broad class of mental operations. Various models have described cognitive control from different focuses, including the Top-down inhibitory model (Aron, 2007), the Working Memory model (Baddeley, 1986), the Supervisory Attentional System (Norman & Shallice, 1980), the

Self-regulatory model (Barkley, 1997) and the Problem-solving model (Zelazo, Carter, Reznick, & Frye, 1997).

Miyake and colleagues (Friedman & Miyake, 2004; Miyake & Friedman, 2012; Miyake et al., 2000) identify three related but separable core aspects of cognitive control: inhibition, mental set shifting, and working memory updating. More recently, Green and Abutalebi (2013) propose the adaptive control hypothesis, stating that cognitive control is divided into eight processes: goal maintenance, conflict monitoring, interference suppression, salient cue detection, selective response inhibition, task disengagement, task engagement, and opportunistic planning. Although different views still exist about the specific subcomponents of cognitive control, it is widely acknowledged that cognitive control as a unitary construct can be separated into some related but independent aspects, which can be measured by different cognitive control tasks. Following this approach, this volume mainly focuses on three aspects: inhibitory control (inhibition), conflict monitoring, and mental set shifting. These aspects have been widely reported related to bilingualism in the literature. *Inhibition* is one's capacity to supersede responses that are prepotent in a given situation. *Conflict monitoring* is one's ability to monitor performance, internal states, and current environment. *Mental set shifting* is one's cognitive flexibility to switch between different tasks or mental states.

1.3 Motivation

Although many studies have found evidence of bilingual advantage in bilinguals compared with their counterpart monolinguals (Bialystok et al., 2005; Bialystok et al., 2004; Bialystok & Viswanathan, 2009; Costa et al., 2009; Prior & Gollan, 2011; Prior & Macwhinney, 2010), quite a few studies have failed to capture positive effects of bilingualism, particularly in behavioral measures among young-adult bilinguals (Bialystok, Craik, & Luk, 2008; Colzato et al., 2008; Hilchey & Klein, 2011; Kousaie & Phillips, 2012a; Luk et al., 2010; Paap & Greenberg, 2013).

For example, in one such study (Paap & Greenberg, 2013), it was concluded that there is no coherence of bilingual cognitive control advantage across different cognitive control tasks and between different studies. In this study, young adult bilinguals and monolinguals were compared in three sub-studies on 15 indicators of executive processing by their performance in the tasks of anti-saccade, Simon, Flanker, and color-shape switching. The results presented no evidence of bilingual advantage and indicated that effects assumed to be indicators of a specific executive process in one task (e.g., inhibitory control in the Flanker task) frequently do not predict individual differences in that same indicator on a related task (e.g., inhibitory control in the Simon task). This study's findings highlight a question central to the most recent research on bilingual advantage – the incoherence of bilingual advantage when examined in different contexts.

The motivation for the current research springs from the need to reinterpret the findings from previous studies that underestimate the incoherence problem, and finds expression in this study's examination of bilingual advantage in different contexts where bilinguals have different bilingual experiences.

1.4 Current Focus

When examining bilingual advantage, most of the previous studies compare cognitive control differences between bilinguals and monolinguals (Bialystok et al., 2005; Bialystok et al., 2004; Bialystok & Viswanathan, 2009; Costa et al., 2009; Prior & Macwhinney, 2010). However, there is at least one crucial shortcoming in this methodology: *The comparison between bilinguals and monolinguals does not distinguish the differences amongst bilinguals, and these differences of bilingual experience may have been a crucial factor in the inability of certain previous studies to find a coherent bilingual advantage.*

Bilingual populations are heterogeneous as there are different kinds, degrees, and dimensions of bilingualism. It should be noted that bilingual advantage is affected by such factors as SES, IQ, gender, and cognitive development, differences which are not related to bilingualism itself. However, bilingual advantage varies amongst bilinguals, and this variance is caused by factors completely independent of those mentioned above – factors inherent in bilingualism itself. The most significant factor is *bilingual experience*. Bilingual experience varies in different contexts; there may be particular patterns or characteristics for the bilinguals in managing the two languages (relative to the general). For example, language proficiency, particularly L2 proficiency, significantly distinguishes bilinguals into different degrees. Moreover, specific language use experience significantly distinguishes bilinguals into different groups. For example, some bilinguals speak L2 more often, whereas others may switch between the two languages more often. These different specific bilingual experiences characterized by uses and patterns may even impact cognitive control among bilinguals.

Therefore, when controlling other factors, investigating cognitive control differences between different bilingual groups who have distinct bilingual experiences may illuminate the nature of bilingual advantage. The current research focuses on how the different bilingual experiences – L2 proficiency, interpreting experience, and public speaking experience – may lead to cognitive control differences among bilinguals.

1.5 Research Overview

In order to examine and characterize bilingual advantage in relation with the heterogeneity of bilingual experience, the current research conducted four experiments.

Experiment One verifies the theory of bilingual advantage in the sense that bilinguals are superior to monolinguals in cognitive control.

Moreover, based on the theory of bilingual advantage, the current research explores the relationship between specific aspects of bilingual experience and cognitive control.

Experiment Two illustrates the relationship between bilingual experience and cognitive control by examining the role of L2 proficiency in enhancing bilinguals' cognitive control.

Experiment Three further clarifies the relationship between bilingual experience and cognitive control by focusing on specific language-use experience, focusing specifically on language interpreting experience.

Experiment Four extends the relationship between bilingual experience and cognitive control to public speaking (L1&L2) experience for bilinguals.

The general contents of this research are outlined below.

Chapter One introduces the importance and necessity of investigating bilingual advantage, by considering the relationship between different bilingual experiences and cognitive control among different bilingual groups. Then, this chapter presents an overview of the main contents in the current research.

Chapter Two provides a general literature review regarding bilingual advantage in cognitive control. Firstly, mechanisms of language processing for bilinguals are analyzed. Secondly, the cognitive impacts of bilingualism are discussed. Thirdly, findings and discussions of bilingual advantage in cognitive control are reviewed.

Chapter Three presents the research rationale and the research questions for the current volume, which aims to prove the existence of bilingual advantage and to further investigate the relationship between specific bilingual experiences and cognitive control enhancement. Designs for four experiments are briefly outlined.

Chapter Four reports an experiment (***Experiment One***) that aims to replicate previous findings that bilinguals have advantage over monolinguals in cognitive control (which is referred to as bilingual advantage) in the Chinese context. A homogeneous group of young-adult unbalanced Chinese-English bilinguals and one group of Chinese counterpart monolinguals were compared in three behavioral tasks: the Flanker task, the Number Stroop task, and the Wisconsin Card Sorting Test (WCST), with the former two tasks measuring inhibition and conflict monitoring and the WCST measuring mental set shifting in cognitive control. In the experiment, bilinguals outperformed monolinguals in the

WCST task measuring mental set shifting, which provides novel evidence to support the existence of bilingual advantage.

Chapter Five reports an experiment (***Experiment Two***) which investigates the relationship between L2 proficiency and cognitive control by comparing two groups of bilinguals with different levels of L2 proficiency. In the experiment, two bilingual groups, distinct in L2 proficiency, were required to perform the same tasks as adopted in *Experiment One*: the Flanker task, the Number Stroop task, and the WCST task. Despite multiple analyses, we were unable to detect any behavioral differences between the two groups differing in L2 proficiency. These results suggest that language proficiency (L2 proficiency) as a complex construct may affect cognitive control in limited or indirect ways.

Chapter Six examines bilingual advantage from one particular bilingual language-use experience: language interpreting. The experiment (***Experiment Three***) compared four groups with the same tasks of Flanker, Number Stroop, and WCST. Two groups without language interpreting experience were used as the control groups, and the other two groups with language interpreting experience were used as the experimental groups. The four groups varied in their L2 proficiency. The results showed that L2 proficiency did not lead to differences but the bilinguals with language interpreting experience significantly outperformed the bilinguals without such experience in the WCST (mental set shifting but not conflict monitoring or inhibiting). Furthermore, the group with greater experience in interpreting performed better than the group with less experience in interpreting.

Chapter Seven reports a further experiment (***Experiment Four***) investigating the relationship between bilingual language-use experience and cognitive control enhancement by focusing on public speaking experience. Two groups of L1/L2 public speaking bilinguals and two groups of controls (one bilingual group, one monolingual group) were tested with the same tasks used in the previous experiments: the Flanker task, the Number Stroop task and the WCST. Results showed that public speaking groups, especially L2 speaking group, performed significantly faster than the control groups in one or more conditions of the Flanker task and the Number Stroop task (conflict monitoring), and groups with higher L2 proficiency performed better than the lower L2 proficiency groups in the WCST (mental set shifting).

Chapter Eight discusses the findings of all the experiments in the current research and relates the findings to the issues and questions in previous literature. The research presented in my volume extends the previously observed advantage for bilinguals relative to monolinguals to the Chinese context and at the same time extends it to the cognitive control differences between bilinguals of heterogeneous experiences.

Finally, ***Chapter Nine*** concludes the current research findings and highlights its contributions and implications in the field.

Chapter 2: Bilingual Advantage

In this literature review, we firstly discuss the mechanisms involved in bilingual language processing, referring to theories and models. Secondly, the review explores both the positive effects and negative consequences of bilingualism based on behavioral and neural results in previous studies. Thirdly, a general report of evidence supporting bilingual advantage in cognitive control is presented. The purpose of this review is two-fold. One is to reveal the broad theoretical background of bilingual advantage and the other is to justify the position of the current research.

2.1 Bilingual Language Processing Mechanism

Bilingual language processing is more complicated than monolingual language processing in three basic areas. Firstly, in language production, bilinguals are similar to monolinguals in the stages of conceptualization, formulation, articulation, and monitoring, but bilinguals are different in that two languages need to be processed instead of one. Secondly, in bilinguals' mind, two languages are activated simultaneously in language processing. Thirdly, since two languages are activated, there is a need for language control mechanism in order to process the target language.

2.1.1 Bilingual Language Processing

Bilingual language processing must be based on the language processing mechanism adopted by monolinguals. Levelt (1989) proposed a classic monolingual language processing model (Figure 1) that consists of a number of processing components, each of which receives a certain kind of input and produces a certain kind of output. The first stage of this model is conceptualizing, which means an intentional activity conceiving of an intention, selecting the relevant information to be expressed. During the processing of concept production, the speaker's constant attention is directed to monitoring what he is saying and how. The product of this conceptualizing is called the preverbal message. In order to encode a preverbal message, the speaker must have the access to both procedural knowledge, which refers to the knowledge of how to realize his intention assertion (such as proposition), and declarative knowledge, which refers to all the structured knowledge of the world and himself (also called encyclopedic knowledge).

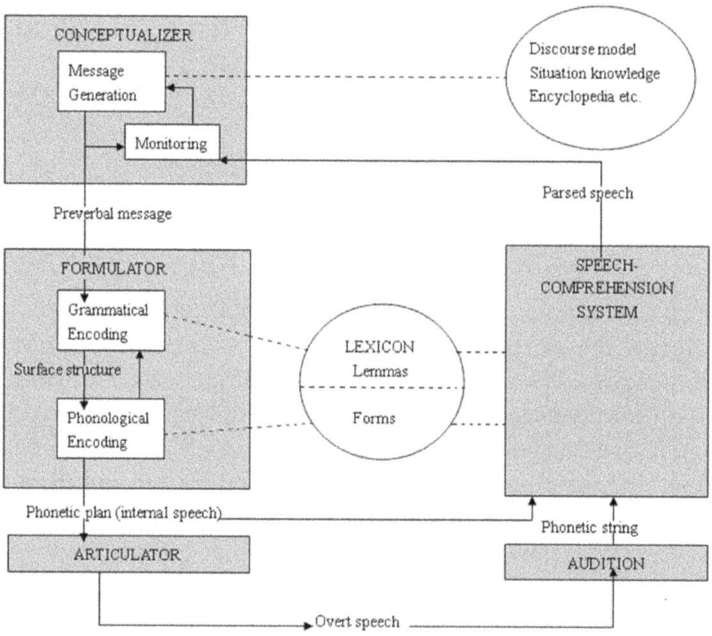

Figure 1. Monolingual Speech Production Model (Levelt, 1989).
(Boxes represent processing components; circle and ellipse represent knowledge stores.)

When the preverbal message is produced, it is sent to Formulator, which accepts fragments of messages as input and produces a phonetic or articulatory plan as output. In the stage of Formulating, there are two steps. First, there is grammatical encoding of the message, which consists of procedures for accessing lemmas, and of syntactic building procedures. With this step done, a surface structure has been produced. Second, there is phonological encoding, which retrieves or builds a phonetic or articulatory plan from lexical form for each lemma and for the utterance as a whole. As a result, a phonetic or articulatory plan is produced.

The phonetic or articulatory plan as input enters the next stage – Articulating, which refers to the motor execution of the phonetic plan by moving the respiratory, the laryngeal, and the supralaryngeal systems. The Articulator retrieves successive chunks of internal speech from the Articulatory Buffer (which may be somewhat ahead of articulatory execution) and unfolds them for execution. The product of articulation is overt speech.

The final part of this model is Self-Monitoring, which is not actually an independent stage just like the previous three stages because self-monitoring happens from the beginning of conceptualizing stage. A speaker listens to himself in different components, including audition processing, speech-comprehension system, parsed speech, internal speech, and the final effect. Speakers not only monitor for meaning but also monitor for linguistic forms according to his intended concept, and if errors are detected, self corrections will be made by returning to the generating model.

Based on Levelt's (1989) Monolingual Speech Model, Kormos (2006) proposed a bilingual speech model (Figure 2), in which she assumes that bilingual speech production is modular in the sense that it consists of separate encoding modules: the conceptualizer, the formulator, and the articulator, which work with their own characteristic input, but parallel processing is also possible because cascading of activations are allowed between the lexical and phonological level of encoding. The production mechanisms are assumed essentially the same in both L1 and L2 and it is also believed that most knowledge stores are shared between L1 and L2. However, in the different stages of language processing, the model assumes that the major difference between L1 and L2 processing originates from the competition of L1 and L2 items, including lexical, phonological, and syntactic encoding procedures.

The first stage is to conceptualize the intended message (preverbal message), which involves the activation of related concepts and the language that is to be used. The message comes from the long-term memory, which consists of several subcomponents: episodic memory, semantic memory including the mental lexicon, the syllabary, and a store for declarative knowledge of L2 rules. L1 and L2 concepts can be identical, shared, or rarely completely separate. When the concept of the message is activated, the language to be chosen is also completed in the stage. It is proposed that language choice is indicated in the form of a language cue, which is to direct the speaker to focus on the intended language.

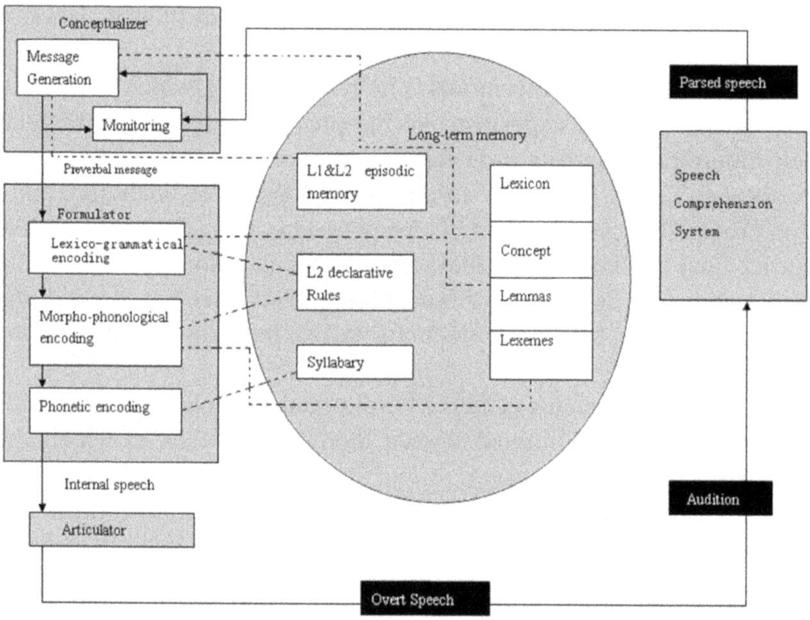

Figure 2. Bilingual Speech Model (Kormos, 2006).

When the preverbal message is ready, it is to be put into the formulating stage, in which lexical, phonological, syntactical, and phonetic encoding are to be processed accordingly. Lexical encoding means the process that matches the conceptual specifications and the language cue with the appropriate lexical entry retrieved from the mental lexicon. Both of L1 and L2 lexicon are potentially activated for selection. In syntactic encoding, two procedures are important. First, the syntactic information such as gender, countability, number, and obligatory complements should be activated. Second, the activated words, phrases, and their syntactic features should be assembled by using the syntactic encoding mechanism. The syntactic information to be activated depends on whether the bilinguals are balanced or not. Balanced bilinguals tend to activate L2 lemmas that are specific for the given L2 entry, while lower L2 speakers tend to activate L2 lemmas of the corresponding L1 item. The next phase is phonological encoding, which activates the phonological form of the words to be encoded, including information such as syllabification, intonation, duration, loudness and pitch etc. It is assumed that the phonological form of non-selected lemmas can also be activated, indicating that L1 and L2 lexemes compete for selection (Colomé, 2001; Costa & Caramazza, 1999). In phonetic encoding, articulatory gestures for syllables are retrieved.

The next stage, termed as articulator, is mainly executive motor action, which utilizes the relevant muscles in a coordinative way to produce the overt speech.

The final component monitoring, which is not exactly a stage because it goes from the beginning through the whole production process, proceeds similarly in both L1 and L2. There are three monitor loops for the production process. The first one is to compare the preverbal message with the speaker's original intention. The second one is to monitor the phonetic plan. The third one is to check, after articulation, whether the generated utterance is correct or intended. There is one important difference between L1 and L2 monitoring, which is that monitoring requires attention. Because attention resources are limited and because L2 is at a lower proficiency level, L2 speech processing needs more attention through different phases and the L2 speakers often have to make conscious decisions what they pay attention to when monitoring.

In the bilingual speech model, Kormos highlighted three differences between L1 and L2 production. The first one is the influence of L1 on L2 processing, which results in the transfer of L1 knowledge in the encoding procedures and the phenomenon of code switching.

The second difference is the incomplete L2 knowledge, which results in the compensation strategies in communication. The third difference is the competition between L1 and L2 items, which is closely relevant to the topic discussed in this volume. The competition between the two languages exerts a significant impact on bilinguals' language processing system and even extends to the general cognitive system. In the following section, I will briefly discuss the theoretical background and findings of competition between L1 and L2 as a result of simultaneous activations of L1 and L2.

2.1.2 Bilingual Lexical Selection

Kormos (2006) put forward an outline of bilingual speech production model, which mentioned that both languages share most conceptual representations and there is competition between L1 and L2. However, the model does not specify two basic questions. The first question is, if the two languages are integrated, how do they compete with each other? The second question is, how do bilinguals select one language over another and at the same time successfully prevent the interference from the non-target language? If bilinguals' two lexicons are integrated, it means that both languages share the same conceptual representations, and then does it mean that the same concept would activate two language representations simultaneously? Then how do bilinguals select the target language in that case? There have been two hypotheses regarding lexical selection mechanism. One hypothesis proposes that the lexical selection process is language specific, which means the selection mechanism considers only the activation levels of lexical nodes of the language-in-use (Roelofs, 1998). The assumption is that a lexicon-external device determines which lexicon is to be consulted, and only lexical nodes in that lexicon are considered for selection. The other hypothesis proposes that a lexicon-external device inhibits or dampens the activation of the lexical items of the language-not-in-use, ensuring that their activation levels are lower than those of the lexical nodes of the language-in-use. This lexical selection mechanism is language non-specific. It considers selection of the lexical items of both languages, and selects the item with the highest activation level (De Bot, 1992; Green, 1998; Poulisse, 1997). The two lexical selection mechanisms are illustrated in Figure 3 and Figure 4.

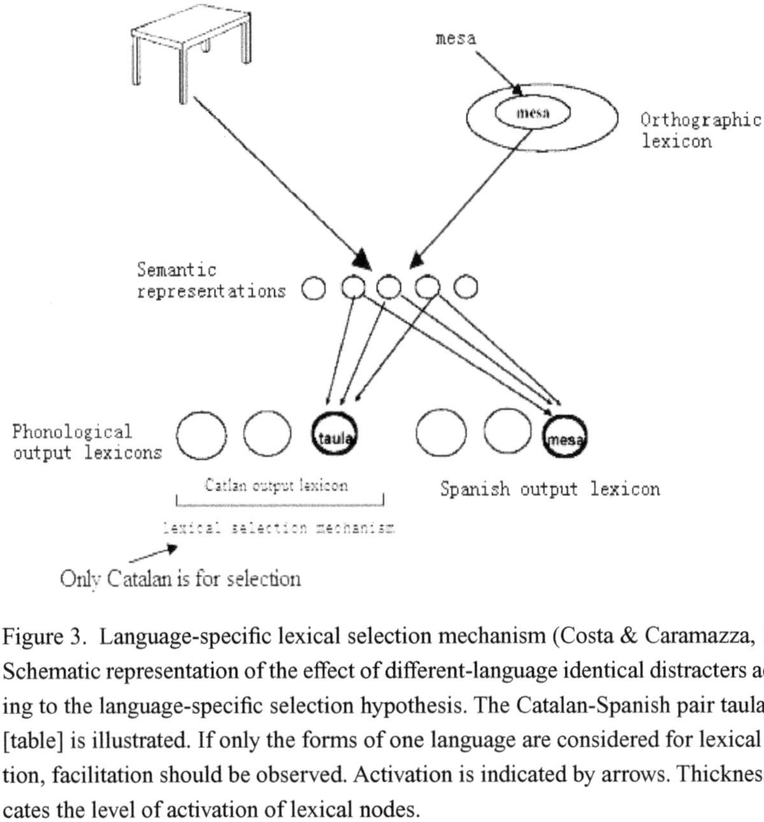

Figure 3. Language-specific lexical selection mechanism (Costa & Caramazza, 1999). Schematic representation of the effect of different-language identical distracters according to the language-specific selection hypothesis. The Catalan-Spanish pair taula-mesa [table] is illustrated. If only the forms of one language are considered for lexical selection, facilitation should be observed. Activation is indicated by arrows. Thickness indicates the level of activation of lexical nodes.

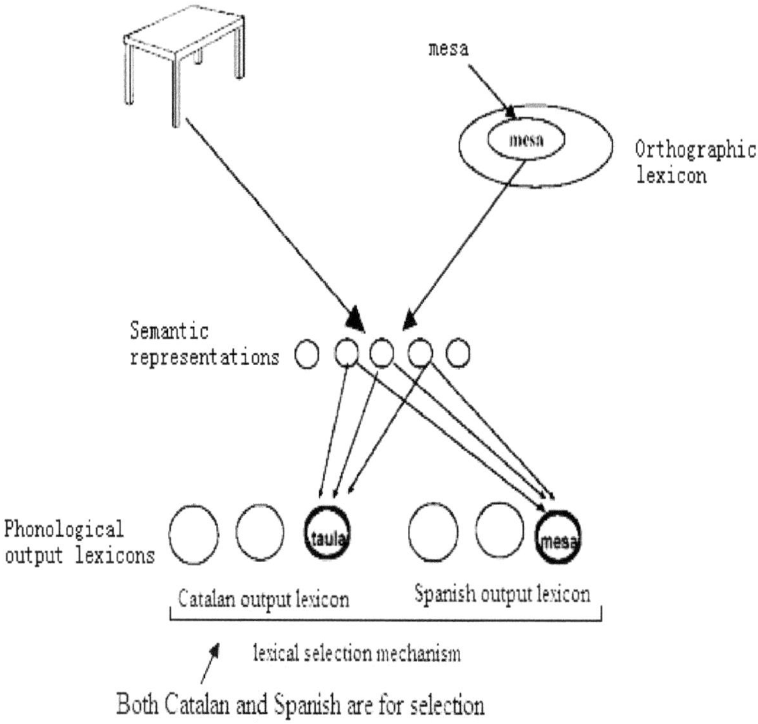

Figure 4. Language non-specific lexical selection mechanism (Costa & Caramazza, 1999). Schematic representation of the effect of different-language identical distracters according to the language non-specific selection hypothesis. If forms of two languages compete for lexical selection, evidence of interference is expected with these pairs. Activation is indicated by arrows. Thickness indicates the level of activation of lexical nodes.

The fact that bilinguals speak either language fluently without much intrusion may give us an intuitive reasoning that we only select the language we want, but experiments tell us that both two languages are potentially activated no matter which language we are using. Empirical studies showed that bilingual word recognition is basically language non-selective, automatic, and its first processing stages might remain unaffected by non-linguistic contextual factors. A large number of studies have confirmed the hypothesis of non-selective activation theory.

Early studies examined bilingual language activation in isolated context. Typical experiment paradigms included lexical decision, word identification, picture naming, and translation recognition etc. in which participants were required to decide or name the target language (a single word or picture). The results showed interference or facilitation by the non-target language. These findings suggested that both meanings of two languages were initially activated (Beauvillain & Grainger, 1987; De Moor, 1998; De Groot, Delmaar, & Lupker, 2000; Schwartz, Kroll, & Diaz, 2007; Blumenfeld & Marian, 2007).

Late studies showed that even in a single language context the interference of non-target language could not be eliminated. Semantic priming has been used in combination with ERPs measurement to examine non-selective bilingual activation. Studies (De Bruijn, Dijkstra, Chwilla, & Schriefers, 2001; Kousaie, 2011) showed that an interlingual homograph primes its meaning in a non-target language, even in the presence of a single word language context. In this paradigm, the amplitude change of N400 component is related to semantic integration (Kutas & Van Petten, 1994). N400 amplitude is related to the match between the target stimulus and a primed or expected stimulus. If a related prime induced smaller N400 amplitude, it meant that the non-target language was activated, relative to when the target stimulus was preceded by an unrelated prime. In another study (Paulmann, Elston-Guttler, Gunter, & Kotz, 2006), it was found that even a global language context (e.g., film context) could not eliminate the influence of non-target language. In a study by Hoshino and Thierry (2011), it was demonstrated that cross-language activation is present even when proficient bilinguals perform a task only in one language. They found that participants named pictures more slowly when distractors were semantically or phonologically related to either the English name of the picture or the Spanish name of the picture than when picture and distractor word were unrelated. These results revealed that lexical activations from both languages compete for selection in the process of L2 speech planning in a predominant L2 context (Hoshino & Thierry, 2011).

In recent neuroimage and ERP studies, researchers have investigated whether the language selection mechanism of bilinguals differs from that of monolinguals. If bilinguals activated two languages simultaneously, their brain activations should be different from those of monolinguals because bilinguals have two active languages in mind. When two languages are activated in bilinguals' brain, how does the selection mechanism work? Studies indicated that language selection is achieved through a neural network involving areas implicated in both general cognitive processes and language processing (Khateb et al., 2007). Language selection means the mechanism that controls two languages is to use at a given moment in a particular context. Studies (Abutalebi et al., 2008) showed that naming in the first language or the weaker second language in the bilingual context (compared to monolingual context) both activated brain areas in the left caudate and anterior cingulate cortex, but the activation of these areas was even more extended when naming in the second weaker language. This finding showed that in bilingual language selection processes in contexts, both languages must remain active by recruiting the brain areas of the left caudate and the anterior cingulate cortexes (ACC), which were distinguished from areas engaged in intra-language selection. Furthermore, in another study using functional magnetic resonance imaging, Parker et al. (2012) found that when bilinguals named pictures or read words aloud, in their native or nonnative language, activation was higher relative to monolinguals in 5 left hemisphere regions: dorsal precentral gyrus, pars triangularis, pars opercularis, superior temporal gyrus, and planum temporale (Parker et al., 2012). These results sufficiently confirmed that bilinguals select two active languages and their language selection mechanism is qualitatively different from that of monolinguals.

The literature presents a general consensus that bilingual lexical access is non-selective in nature: the non-target language can interfere with the target language during production or comprehension, even in completely monolingual contexts. This review provides sufficient evidence in support of the view that bilingual language activation is non-selective – a bilingual's two languages are activated simultaneously, both receptively and productively, both in isolated situations and in global single-language contexts. Thus bilinguals cannot completely 'turn off' one language – both are activated in parallel and can interact with each other. This non-selective language activation process thus becomes a unique mechanism for bilinguals. Therefore, since two languages are activated simultaneously, regardless of the language context, it is evident that the way in which bilinguals manage to articulate only the language they want to speak is critical to bilingual language processing. There must be a mechanism by which attention can be directed to the target language and by which the non-target language can be inhibited. In the following section, I will present literature concerning this language control mechanism. It is this language control mechanism that guarantees the successful language processing for bilinguals.

2.1.3 Language Control Mechanism

Several language control models in bilingualism research have been proposed to explain how bilinguals control and select languages (van Heuven & Dijkstra, 2010). In the following section, I will present a few of the models related to language control and selection.

Being a bilingual means there must be two linguistic subsystems in one's mind. The two language systems somehow must specify which one of the stored units belongs to one linguistic subsystem and which one belongs to the other. Several proposals have been advanced for this purpose. The first one was called "subset", which means that the elements of each language are embedded in a separate network of strongly interconnected elements within bilingual memory (Grosjean, 1997; Paradis, 1981, 2004). The second one was called "language nodes", which means the form representations of all L1 words are connected to the L1 language node, and the form representations of all L2 words are connected to the L2 language node (Dijkstra & van Heuven, 1998; Dijkstra & van Heuven, 2002). The third one was called "language tag", which means a piece of information that specifies that this particular lemma belongs to L1 or L2 (Green, 1998; Poulisse, 1997).

Researchers have proposed several models of bilingual language control. The bilingual language control models provide insights into the nature of bilingual advantage. Penfield and Roberts (1959) advanced "language switch mechanism" to regulate and control the different use of languages. They proposed that there is an effective and automatic switch that allows each individual to turn from one language to another. Bilinguals including infants have the capacity to switch languages according to the language characteristics of the interlocutor (Penfield & Roberts, 1959). Macnamara and Kushnir (1971) proposed "input switch" to explain why bilinguals took longer to read mixed-language text passages when compared to single-language passages, even though the passages were otherwise equivalent in length and complexity. In this theory, when a bilingual person encounters a switch of one language, the comprehension mechanism of that language was switched off and the mechanism of the other language was switched on (Macnamara & Kushnir, 1971). This theory was criticized because it assumed that bilinguals' two languages were not simultaneously activated (Moreno et al., 2008). Another model was called "monolingual-bilingual mode continuum model" put forward by Grosjean (1985, 1997). The model proposed that bilinguals move along a continuum where one extreme represents a completely monolingual mode while the other end depicts a fully bilingual mode, depending on the situation (Grosjean, 1985, 1997). However, this model did not describe how bilinguals move from one end to the other, and the full independence of monolingual mode was still questionable.

The widely accepted models of language control were based on a prerequisite that language activation is non-selective. There are two models that directly explain language control for bilinguals. The first one is the BIA+ model, which is an integration of bottom-up and top-down nature of language processing. The second one is the Inhibitory Control model, which considers language control as similar to general cognitive control, and the control is achieved through task schemas, word selection, and inhibiting irrelevant lemmas. We will explain these two models in the following sections.

2.1.3.1 The BIA+ Model

The Bilingual Interactive Activation Plus (BIA+) is a model for understanding the process of bilingual language comprehension and consists of two interactive subsystems: the word identification subsystem and task/decision subsystem (van Heuven & Dijkstra, 2010). It is the successor of the Bilingual Interactive Activation (BIA) model (Figure 5) (Dijkstra, van Heuven, & Grainger, 1998; Grainger & Dijkstra, 1992) which was updated in 2002 to include phonologic and semantic lexical representations, revise the role of language nodes, and specify the purely bottom-up nature of bilingual language processing.

In the BIA model, language nodes are supposed to function in a way that inhibits the non-target language. Their top-down influence is not thought to alter the early activation of words in each of the two languages but to increase the later likelihood of selecting a word from the intended language (Dijkstra & van Heuven, 2002).

On the contrary, the BIA+ Model distinguishes between a word identification system and a task/decision system (Figure 6) and proposes an integrated bilingual lexicon, in which the words in a target language are selected by means of a higher-level control system.

Within the word identification system, orthographic inputs activate associated phonological and semantic representations, as well as associated language nodes which act as tags specifying a word's language membership. These language nodes are connected directly to lexical form representations, so the activation of language nodes depends on the activation of other linguistic representations. As representations from different languages are activated, the word identification system collects the relative activation and passes this information to the task/decision system, which achieves response selection by weighing the relative activation of language node information from the word identification system and making a decision based on the specific task goal.

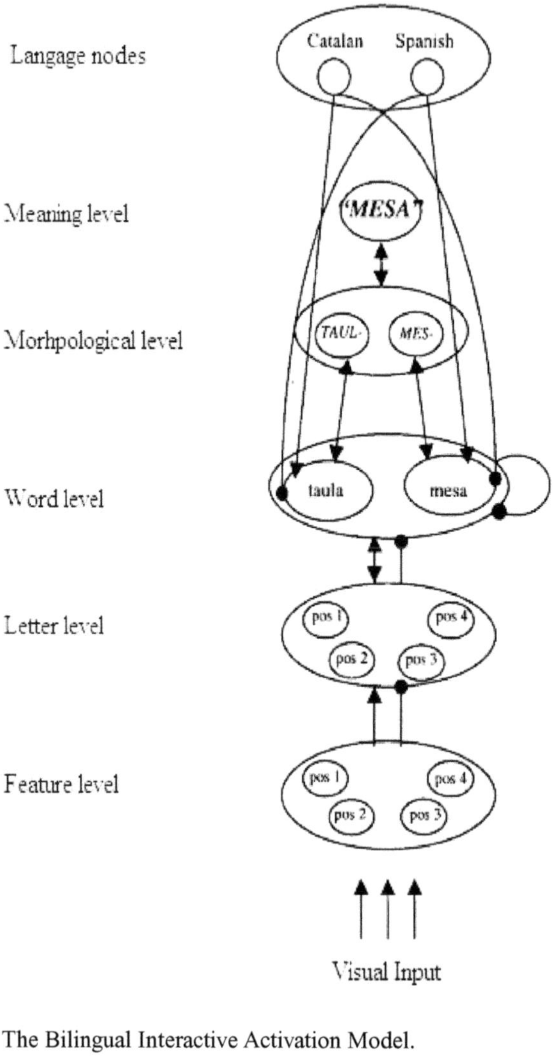

Figure 5. The Bilingual Interactive Activation Model.

BIA model. Arrow heads indicate excitatory connections; black-filled circles indicate inhibitory connections. Though only four positions for features and letters are represented, the model is not limited to the recognition of four-letter words.

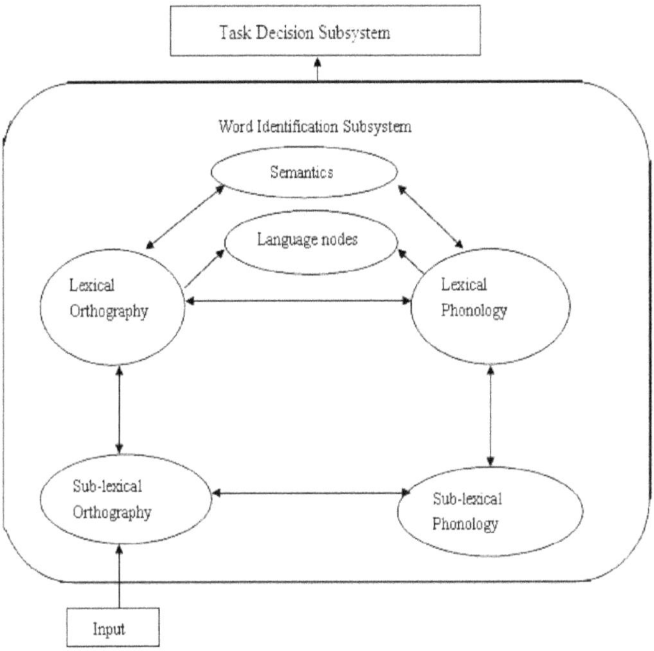

Figure 6. A flow chart representation of the BIA+ model for bilingual language processing including the word identification and task/decision subsystems.

2.1.3.2 The Inhibitory Control Model

The Inhibitory Control Model (ICM) (Green, 1998) is a model explicitly addressing bilingual language control (Figure 7). Previous studies on bilingual advantage are mostly stimulated by this theory. According to this model, language control is akin to general cognitive control. The realization of control relies on three levels. The first level deals with the competition of language task schemas for control of the target language. When a language task schema is specified (e.g. L1 word production), the schema will regulate the output of lexical-semantic system and inhibit the irrelevant schema until the goal is achieved. Inhibitory links within and between the language task schemas ensure that the task goals of a higher-level 'supervisory attentional system' (SAS) are met. The second level involves selection of word. Words are selected according to language tag and only word of the target language will be selected. The third level concerns the very important function of inhibiting irrelevant lemmas. Lemmas of incorrect tags will be suppressed.

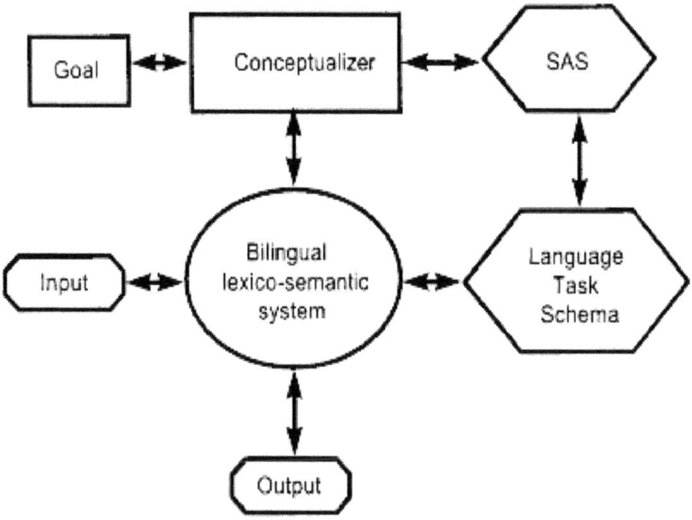

Figure 7. The Inhibitory Control Model (Green, 1998), SAS – supervisory attentional system.

To illustrate, when a bilingual speaker intends to speak in L2, the SAS conceptualizes this goal and then modulates the activation of the language task schemas of the L1 and L2. As the L2 is the goal, both language task schemas inhibit lemmas with an L1 language tag. Language control in the ICM model is thus cross-linguistically inhibitory (i.e. is exerted by the target L2 task schema over the non-target L1 task schema) and self-inhibitory (i.e. within the L1 language task schema).

Evidence for the Inhibitory Control Model (Green, 1986; Green, 1998) comes from studies of different types. The most popular techniques for studying language control in bilinguals are the picture-word interference paradigm, the "language-switching paradigm", and language-specific property effect (Kroll, Bobb, Misra, & Guo, 2008). In the following paragraphs, I will briefly review the investigations that have adopted each of these approaches.

In the standard version of picture-word interference (PWI) paradigm, a picture is presented, followed by a distractor word at a variable

SOA with respect to the presentation of the picture. Participants are required to name the picture while ignoring the distractor. The typical result of this task is that words semantically related to the picture are named slower because of interference and words phonologically / orthographically related to the picture are named faster because of facilitation (La Heij, vander Heijden, & Schreuder, 1985; Lupker, 1979, 1982). In the bilingual version of the task, the distractor words are from the non-target language, either semantically related to the picture, or phonologically/orthographically related to the picture. This bilingual version produced similar results: interference and facilitation, respectively (Costa, Miozzo, & Caramazza, 1999).

In studies using a language switching paradigm, the bilingual participants have to switch between their two languages, mostly randomly but sometimes in a regular pattern. The purpose of this task is to find out what happens in their minds during switch trials and non-switch trials. The critical dependent variable in language switching studies was the time it took to switch between languages – switch cost. Studies show that switching from a second language to a native language takes larger switch costs than switching from a native language to a second language (Filippi, Karaminis, & Thomas, 2013; Meuter & Allport, 1999). This asymmetry of switch cost was taken as evidence for the active inhibition of a native language (dominant language) during naming in a second language (non-dominant language). Meuter and Allport (1999) explained the asymmetry of switch costs in terms of suppression that the dominant task must be actively suppressed in order to prevent interference with the non-dominant task, so when switching to the dominant task, the active suppression of the dominant task on the preceding non-dominant trial persists to disrupt processing the subsequent trial. However, the asymmetry of switch cost may disappear as experiment tasks or participants vary. Some studies (Costa, Santesteban, & Ivanova, 2006; Finkbeiner, Almeida, Janssen, & Caramazza, 2006) also found that inhibition operates in bilinguals during language switching, but they suggested that asymmetric switch cost might be due to bivalent stimuli and that in highly proficient bilinguals switch cost asymmetry might disappear. A recent study by Gollan and Feirreira (2007) also reported no symmetric switch costs when switches were under participants' own control (Gollan & Ferreira, 2007). However, the symmetry or asymmetry of switch costs in all itself may not reveal the means of language selection. In both cases, inhibition is required to overcome the activation of competitors from the non-target language when bilinguals produce words in one of their languages (Kroll et al., 2008).

The third approach of evidence comes from a paradigm using a language-specific property to determine whether non-target language is available or activated for selection. A number of studies examined cross-language shared words that are phonologically or orthographically similar (e.g. cognates) and found that bilinguals name pictures whose names are cognates faster than pictures whose names are non-cognates (Costa, Caramazza, & Sebastian-Galles, 2000; Hoshino & Kroll, 2008). This suggests that the phonological properties of the non-target language are active during the naming of intended language, which is only present for bilinguals. In Hoshino and Kroll (2008)'s study, the target language and non-target languages did not share similar script (Japanese-English), but they also observed cognate facilitation in picture naming (Hoshino & Kroll, 2008).

All the results from previous studies by the three typical approaches suggest that inhibitory control is required to overcome the activation of competing language lemmas from the non-target language. It has been proved that inhibitory process must be at work to modulate cross-language activity so that the correct target language could be produced (Kousaie, 2011).

2.2 Cognitive Impact of Bilingualism

The previous section demonstrates that for bilinguals both languages are activated in their language processing, and language control is needed in order to select the target language. The regular use of two languages by bilingual individuals has been shown to have a broad impact on language and cognitive functioning (Bialystok et al., 2009; Kar, Khare, & Dash,

2011; Peal & Lambert, 1962; Pearson et al., 1993; Schweizer, Craik, & Bialystok, 2013). In the following paragraphs, I will present literature concerning the impact of bilingualism on language and cognitive functioning, both in terms of disadvantages and advantages.

2.2.1 Bilingual Disadvantages

Some studies showed that speaking more than one language might cause disadvantages (Bialystok et al., 2009; Bialystok, Craik, & Luk, 2012). The fact that monolinguals and bilinguals have different language processing system and that the two languages are non-selectively activated in a bilingual mind thus causing interference between the two languages poses a possibility that bilinguals need more effort to manage languages in production and comprehension. As might be expected, having two (or more) languages to choose from consequently impedes (or, in some cases, facilitates) language processing.

In the study of cognitive development, as mentioned earlier, it was believed that learning two languages might cause detrimental effects upon bilingual children's intelligence and mental state (Saer, 1923; Smith, 1923). In Smith (1923)'s study, for example, two levels (standard III, standard VII) of child monolinguals and bilinguals completed several tests, including writing an essay in a 15-minute time period and forming words from six letters. The results found that for free composition monolinguals had an advantage over bilinguals in standard III level children, and the advantage was even greater in standard VII level, whereas the advantage was observed only in standard VII level between monolinguals and bilinguals for the word forming test.

For other aspects, it has been reported that throughout the lifespan, bilinguals have a smaller vocabulary size in each language compared with monolinguals and are reported slower in lexical processing (including both comprehension and production), although the vocabulary size measure and standard is somewhat controversial. Studies have generally reported negative effect of bilingualism on lexical measures. Several researchers have found that bilinguals show lower levels of receptive vocabulary than do their monolingual peers. Ben-Zeev showed a 10-point deficit on the Peabody Picture Vocabulary Test (PPVT) for

Hebrew-English bilingual 7-year-olds (Ben-Zeev, 1977). Rosenblum and Pinker found bilingual 5-year-olds scored 26 points lower than did their monolingual counterparts on the PPVT (Rosenblum & Pinker, 1983). And later a careful investigation examining how many words children between 8 and 30 months old knew in each language confirmed that, on average, this number was smaller in each language for bilingual children than for monolingual learners of that language (Pearson et al., 1993). As mentioned earlier, Bialystok et al. (2010) provided a clearer illustration of the relative vocabulary size of monolinguals and bilinguals. They measured the receptive vocabulary of over 1,700 children between the ages of 3 and 10 years old. The results showed that at every age studies, the mean standard score on the English Peabody Picture Vocabulary Test (PPVT) of receptive vocabulary was reliably higher for monolinguals than for bilinguals (Bialystok et al., 2010).

In addition, bilinguals are reported to process their L2 in a slower speed when compared to native speakers of that language. It is quite understandable that bilinguals have a lower-proficiency in L2, thus in a weaker or less-dominant situation. It is proposed that the strength of connections between words and concepts are modulated by experience and practice (Lovett, 2002). The lower proficiency in L2 means that bilinguals have less experience and practice with L2. Thus there is weaker connections strength between words and concepts in the L2 language system. Weaker strength between nodes in the L2 language system will therefore accumulate activation more slowly, taking longer to reach the threshold and resulting in 'slower' language processing. Evidence comes from a range of tasks demonstrating that bilinguals experience difficulties and delays in lexical processing in their L2 (Runnqvist, Strijkers, Sadat, & Costa, 2011; van Heuven & Dijkstra, 2010). Bilinguals experience more tip-of-the-tongue (ToT) states than monolinguals when naming pictures in their L2, demonstrating word-finding difficulties (Moreno et al., 2008; Pyers, Gollan, & Emmorey, 2009). Bilinguals also produce their L2 or less-dominant language more slowly than monolinguals in picture naming (Gollan, Montoya, Cera, & Sandoval, 2008). Some studies using EEG provides fine-grained neural evidence that L2 processing is delayed. The L2 experiences delays in higher-level semantic and syntactic ERP components such as the N400 and P600 (Moreno et al., 2008).

Similarly, bilinguals also produce L1 more slowly when compared to L1 native speakers (Finkbeiner, Gollan, & Caramazza, 2006). It has been proposed, as mentioned above, that bilinguals use each of their languages including L1 less often, compared to monolinguals. Therefore, the reduced frequency of using L1 consequently lead to weaker connection strength between words and concepts, which slows the speed of lexical retrieval in language processing. In other words, bilingual lexical access is slower than that of monolinguals even when both groups are performing in their native language (Gollan et al., 2008). Furthermore, EEG studies (Ardal, Donald, Meuter, Muldrew, & Luce, 1990; Proverbio, Čok, & Zani, 2002) also reported that bilinguals were slower to make grammaticality judgments on sentences in their native language than monolinguals were and bilinguals reported a small but significant delay in the N400 response to semantically-anomalous sentences for bilinguals when performing in their L1 compared to monolinguals.

Furthermore, reliable differences between monolinguals and bilinguals have been reported when they perform the verbal fluency task. In the task, both bilinguals and monolinguals are asked to generate as many words as possible within 60 seconds, determined either by the category (semantic fluency) or the initial letter of the word (phonological fluency), in which category fluency is strongly indicative of vocabulary size (e.g., how many types of fruit can you name?). The results showed that bilinguals generate fewer words than monolinguals in semantic fluency (category) (Linck, Kroll, & Sunderman, 2009; Luo, Luk, & Bialystok, 2010).

In summary, one prominent negative impact of bilingualism on cognition is a processing delay or slower speed on a range of linguistic levels, such as lexical retrieval in word recognition and production, semantic and syntactic integration. Specifically, this processing delay or slower speed is manifested particularly in L2 processing, while there is also evidence indicating slower processing of L1, compared to native speakers of each language. As a result of slowed speed in both L1 and

L2 language processing, bilinguals produce fewer words in verbal fluency task related to vocabulary size.

However, in contrast to the disadvantages relevant to bilingual language processing, managing two or more languages in the brain confers cognitive benefits or advantages among bilinguals. I will present an overview of the issue in the next section.

2.2.2 Bilingual Advantages

Keeping two (or more) languages working in the brain causes interference in language processing, but the necessity to manage two languages in an efficient way brings about cognitive benefits in different categories, which mainly include metalinguistic awareness, learning ability, creativity, and cognitive control.

Metalinguistic Awareness

Metalinguistic awareness is the ability to attend to, and reflect upon, the properties of a language. Metalinguistic awareness is often assessed using tasks of phonological and syntactical awareness. Tests of phonological awareness usually require the analysis of sounds in words, whereas tests of syntactical awareness assess children's understanding of the form and grammar of utterances. Previous research has shown that metalinguistic awareness may be enhanced in bilingual children, because learning two languages may require one to focus on the properties of both languages. Bilinguals may have a stronger awareness of the arbitrary relationship between language form and meaning. For example, bilinguals may be more acceptable to sentences like "Apples grow on noses" (Suppose English is one of the two languages), compared with English monolinguals (Bialystok, 1987; Cummins, 1978). It is proposed that bilingual children consistently outperform monolinguals on some metalinguistic tasks. Rather than attributing this advantage to privileged access to a domain of knowledge, however, the benefit is traced to a specific cognitive process that develops more readily in bilingual children. This control process of attention is central to certain metalinguistic problems, and it is in solving these problems that bilingual children excel (Bialystok, 2001). A recent study (Bialystok,

Peets, Moreno, & Sylvain, 2012) examined metalinguistic awareness in children who were becoming bilingual in an immersion education program with a purpose to determine at what point in emerging bilingualism the metalinguistic advantages may appear. Participants were 124 children in second and fifth grades who were enrolled in either a French immersion or a regular English program. The results from tasks measuring morphological awareness, syntactic awareness, and verbal fluency demonstrated the gradual emergence of changes in metalinguistic concepts associated with bilingualism over a period of about 5 years. Bilinguals are also reported more efficient at monitoring linguistic errors compared to monolingual counterparts (Davidson & Indefrey, 2011; Yudes, Macizo, Morales, & Bajo, 2012). However, not all studies examining metalinguistic abilities found improved performance for bilinguals. This can be explained by a range of factors related to bilingualism, such as the nature of the task, degree of reliance on executive function resources, similarity between the two languages, etc.

Learning Ability

A few studies have examined whether bilingualism may have effect upon novel learning. In a study examining the cognitive control mechanisms in adult English speaking monolinguals compared to early sequential Spanish-English bilinguals during the initial stages of novel word learning, it was found that monolinguals activated a broader set of cortical control regions associated with higher-level cognitive processes, including the supplementary motor area (SMA), anterior cingulate (ACC), and dorsolateral prefrontal cortex (DLPFC), as well as the caudate, implicated in cognitive control of language, while bilinguals recruited a more localized subcortical network that included the putamen, associated more with motor control of language. These results suggest that the experience managing multiple languages may differentiate the learning strategy used by bilinguals compared to monolinguals in the early stages of novel word learning (Bradley, King, & Hernandez, 2012). In another study (Bartolotti & Marian, 2012), monolinguals and bilinguals were taught an artificial language designed to elicit between-language competition. Partial activation of interlingual competitors was assessed with eye-tracking and mouse-tracking during a word recognition task in the novel language. Eye-tracking results showed that monolinguals looked at competitors more than bilinguals, and for a longer duration of time. Mouse-tracking results showed that monolinguals' mouse movements were attracted to native-language competitors, whereas bilinguals overcame competitor interference by increasing the activation of target items. These results indicate that bilingualism may facilitate learning a new language.

Creativity

Studies also propose that the experience of managing two languages contributes to creative abilities. One of the earliest studies surveyed twenty-four such reports and found that twenty of these reports showed that bilinguals performed better than monolinguals on creativity (Ricciardelli, 1992). There have been more recent studies that reported this bilingual advantage on creativity. For example, in one study, high-proficient bilinguals and low-proficient bilinguals were compared when they performed creativity tasks tapping into convergent and divergent thinking. The results showed a bilingual advantage among the high-proficient bilinguals for convergent thinking but not divergent thinking, which suggests that bilingualism should not be related to "creativity" as a unitary concept but, rather, to the specific processes and mechanisms that underlie creativity (Hommel, Colzato, Fischer, & Christoffels, 2011). In another study (Kharkhurin, 2011), it was found that linguistically advanced bilinguals demonstrated greater abilities to produce original and useful ideas and to think beyond standard categories in creative problem-solving. The author identified two mechanisms of selective attention as contributors. Firstly, the inhibition of irrelevant information seemed to enhance the capacity to produce original and useful ideas. Secondly, the facilitation of relevant information was likely to boost the ability to activate a multitude of unrelated concepts and work through the concepts already activated. The possible effect of bilingualism on creativity has also been found in nonmathematical and mathematical problem solving. In one such study (Leikin, 2012), all children (three groups: bilinguals from bilingual kindergarten, bilinguals from monolingual kindergarten, monolinguals) performed the Picture Multiple Solution task on general creativity and the Creating Equal Number task on mathematical creativity. The results reveal that both early bilingualism and some form of bilingual education seem to influence the children's general and mathematical creativity.

Cognitive Control
The interaction between bilingualism and the cognitive system is best manifested in an advantage in cognitive control that generalizes beyond language processing to other aspects of cognitive functioning. When we refer to bilingual advantage, we mean primarily advantages in cognitive control. As already mentioned, earlier studies suggest that learning two languages is detrimental to children's cognitive development because children have to learn two vocabularies, two grammars, or even two cultures, which in the end causes strong interference in language processing (Saer, 1923). This negative view was initially questioned by Peal and Lambert (1962). In their study, a few intelligence tests were given to French-English bilingual children and English monolinguals. It was expected that the performance of monolinguals and bilinguals would be similar on nonverbal intelligence and bilinguals might perform lower on verbal intelligence tests. However, to their surprise, bilinguals were better than monolinguals on almost all the tests, including nonverbal tests. A further analysis suggests that there is no significant difference between bilinguals and monolinguals on spatial-perceptual abilities tests, but there is a significant advantage for bilinguals in tests requiring symbol manipulation and reorganization (Peal & Lambert, 1962). This finding initiated a tide of tremendous research aiming to find evidence in support of bilingual advantage. Up to now, there have been numerous studies with this goal. I will review the most representative ones in the next section.

2.3 Bilingual Advantage in Cognitive Control

Cognitive control, as already mentioned, refers to the ability to control the processes that allow information processing or behavior to change flexibly according to different goals. Cognitive control includes a broad class of aspects, including inhibition, conflict monitoring, and mental set shifting, and working memory updating. It has been widely reported that bilinguals have advantage in performing cognitive control tasks relative to monolinguals (see Bialystok et al., 2009 for a review). However, before going into the review of bilingual advantage in cognitive control, a clear understanding of how cognitive control can be operationally measured is a prerequisite to evaluate the validity of relevant studies of bilingual advantage in cognitive control.

2.3.1 Measurement of Cognitive Control

Different paradigms have been used to measure cognitive control abilities in different aspects. Here we introduce only the paradigms measuring *inhibition, conflict monitoring, and mental set shifting*, as these aspects have been reported mostly related to bilingualism in literature. These paradigms generally can be categorized into two types. That is, behavioral assessment and neurological assessment. In the current research, we will adopt behavioral measures.

2.3.1.1 Behavioral Assessment

Measuring Inhibition and Conflict Monitoring

In behavioral assessment, some typical conflict resolution paradigms such as the Stroop (Stroop, 1935), the Simon (Simon, 1969), and the Flanker (Eriksen & Eriksen, 1974) are widely used. These paradigms assess *inhibitory control (inhibition)* required to ignore a conflicting cue in order to respond to a target cue, in which participants are required to respond to one stimulus stimulation while suppressing or ignoring another. For example, in the Flanker Task, which refers to a set of response inhibition tests used in cognitive psychology to assess the ability to suppress responses that are inappropriate in a particular context, a central stimulus (usually an arrow, or a letter) is flanked by non-target stimuli. Congruent trials contain facilitating information (flanked by the same directional response as the target), and incongruent trials contain conflicting information (flanked by the opposite directional response as the target), while neutral trials generally contain no conflicting or facilitating information (e.g. an arrow flanked by lines or squares). It is found that response times are slower for incongruent stimuli than for congruent stimuli (Figure 8).

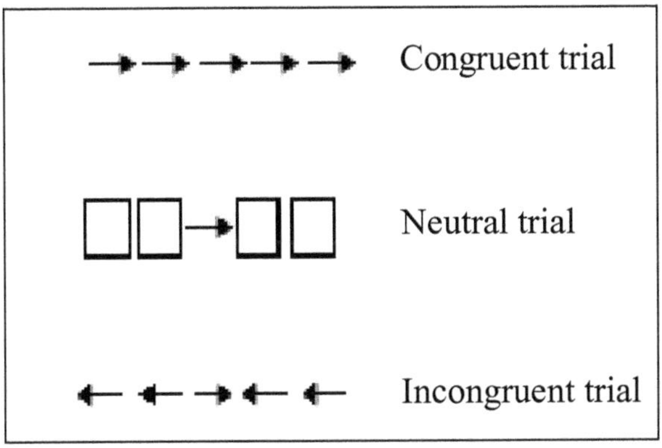

Figure 8. Example of Flanker trials.

Another common conflict paradigm, particularly in bilingualism research, is the Simon task (Figure 9), in which a colored square is presented peripherally on the screen and participants indicate its color using one of two hands (e.g. left hand for blue, right hand for red). In incongruent conditions, the hand required for response differs from the laterality of stimulus presentation (e.g. a red square, requiring a right-hand response, presented on the left side of the screen). Congruent conditions consist of converging spatial and response information, whereas neutral conditions contain no conflicting or converging information.

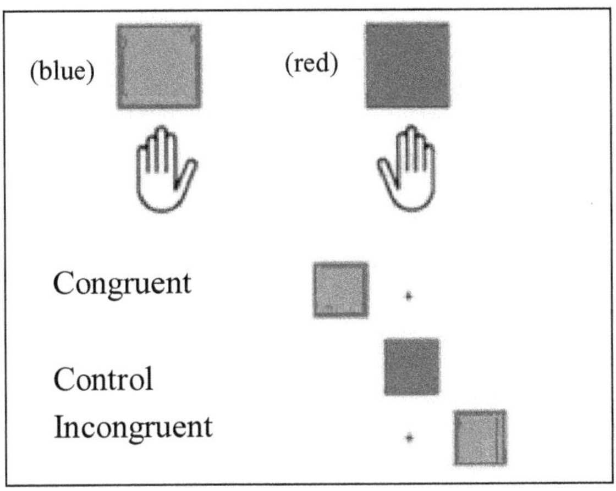

Figure 9. Example of the Simon task (Coderre, 2012).

In a traditional Stroop task, participants are presented with color words printed in colored ink and must overcome the highly automatic reading process in order to name the color of the ink (Figure 10). In incongruent condition, the word meaning and the printed word color conflicts (e.g. the word red printed in blue ink). In congruent condition, the word meaning and the printed word color matches (e.g. the word red printed in red ink). In neutral condition, the word is replaced by non-word symbol strings in colored ink (e.g. %%%% in red).

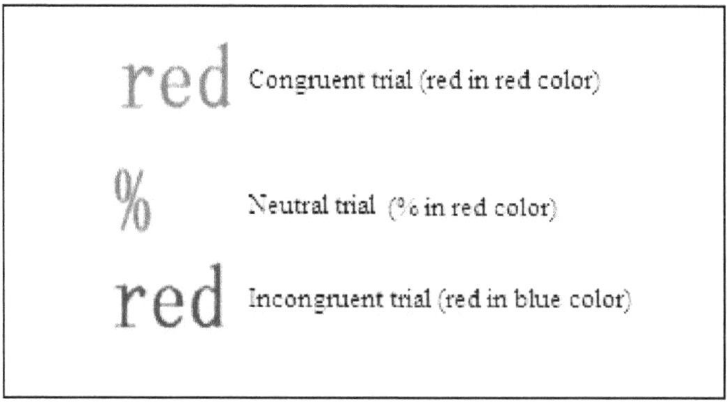

Figure 10. Example of congruent, neutral, and incongruent stimuli, respectively, in the Stroop task.

In all these cognitive control tasks, participants often respond more slowly in incongruent conditions because incongruence consumes additional time to overcome the conflicting information, but participants respond more quickly in congruent conditions because congruence facilitates the processing of converging information. In neutral condition, participants respond generally between the incongruent and congruent conditions in speed because the neutral condition does not generate any interference or facilitation. The difference between the incongruent and congruent conditions, termed the 'conflict effect' (Stroop/Simon/Flanker effect), is often reported to indicate the efficiency to suppress interference from irrelevant conflicting information (inhibition), whereas overall RTs in each condition is reportedly to indicate the functioning of conflict monitoring in conditions where participants need to continuously monitor the appropriate response (Costa et al., 2009).

Measuring Mental Set Shifting

In measuring mental set shifting, A-not-B task, Task Switch, Dimensional Change Card Sorting Test, Multiple Classification Card Sorting Task, and Wisconsin Card Sorting Test are commonly used paradigms. Task Switch and Wisconsin Card Sorting Task are typical examples. Task switching (Jersild, 1927), which is credited to Jersild (1927) who had students time themselves working through a list of items, either repeating one task or alternating between two, is an experimental research paradigm frequently used in cognitive and experimental psychology. It is mainly used to investigate executive functions of cognitive flexibility or set-shifting. It consists of swapping between different tasks or rules. This ability allows a person to rapidly and efficiently adapt to different situations.

In a task-switching experiment, subjects are first pre-trained on two or more simple tasks afforded by a set of stimuli. Each task requires attention to, and classification of, a different element or attribute of the stimulus, or retrieval from memory or computation of a different property of the stimulus. Then, a stimulus is presented on each of a series of trials and the subject performs one of the tasks. There are several methods for telling the subject which task to perform, but in all cases the task sometimes changes from one trial to the next, and sometimes does not. Thus, we can examine performance on trials when the task changes for evidence of extra processing demands that are associated with the need to reconfigure task-set (Monsell, 2003). A task set is typically assumed to include a representation of a task goal (e.g., attend to stimulus color), a set of task-relevant stimuli (e.g., red and blue), a set of possible responses (e.g., press a left or a right key), and a mapping of stimuli – or stimulus categories – to responses (Monsell, 1996).

For example, in a color-shape task switch, subjects might switch between a color discrimination task (e.g. red, green) and a shape discrimination task (e.g. circle, triangle), in which the two dimensions appear by trials, and are mapped onto dedicated response keys. Subjects need to rely on a task set when they are required to respond to stimulus color or shape. That is, when subjects switch between colors and shapes, they need to switch between competing task sets (Figure 11). Usually two measures of executive control can be computed. Switching costs (also called specific or local switching costs) are defined as the difference in response times between switch and non-switch trials in the mixed-task blocks, and are thought to reflect the difficulty in switching from one task set to another. Mixing costs (also called general or global switching costs) are termed as the difference in response times between single-task blocks and non-switch trials in the mixed-task blocks. Mixing costs may indicate the activation of global sustained control mechanisms necessary for maintaining two competing task/response sets, for monitoring the task cued or for a process of task decision on each trial (Prior & Macwhinney, 2010).

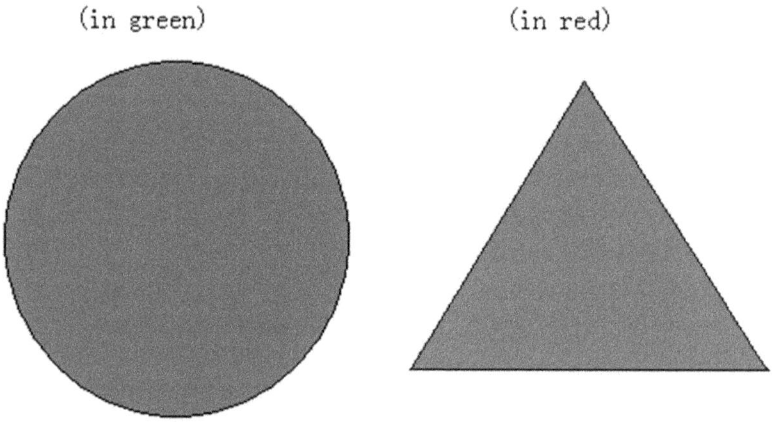

Figure 11. Example stimuli of color-shape task switch.

In Wisconsin Card Sorting Test (Figure 12), which is more complex than color-shape switching, there are three dimensions to switch. WCST consists of four keycards and 128 response cards with geometric figures that vary according to three perceptual dimensions (color, shape, or number).The task requires subjects to find the correct classification principle by trial and error and examiner feed-back. Once the subject chooses the correct rule they must maintain this sorting principle (or set) across changing stimulus conditions while ignoring the other – now irrelevant – stimulus dimensions. After a number of (e.g. 8 or 9) consecutive correct matches, the classification principle changes without warning, demanding a flexible shift inset. The WCST is usually not timed and sorting continues until all cards are sorted or a maximum of correct sorting criteria have been reached. Many authors normally rely on no more than two or three scores as an index of subject's performance, including: number of categories completed, number of perseverative errors, and number of non-perseverative errors (Nyhus & Barcelo, 2009; Yudes, Macizo, & Bajo, 2011).

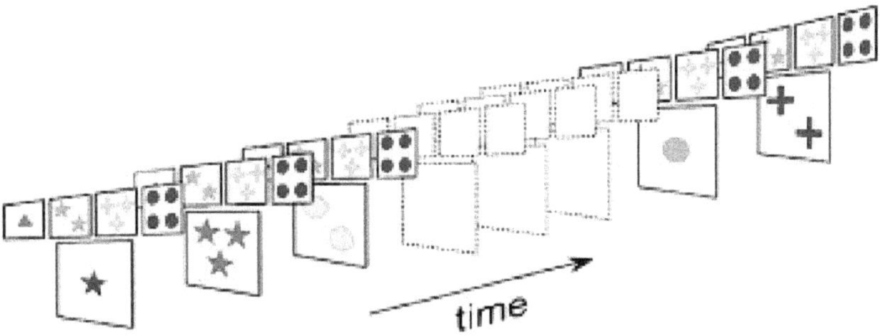

Figure 12. Example procedure of the WCST (Nyhus & Barcelo, 2009).

2.3.1.2 Neurocognitive Assessment

ERPs Measurement

The method of event-related potentials (ERPs) allows us to examine the time course of language (task) processing from the perspective of neurocognitive mechanism with sensitive millisecond resolution. Cognitive control tasks typically generate two conflict-related components: N200, an early negativity (around 200 ms or later post-stimulus) in the incongruent condition, and LPC (late positive component), a later positivity in the incongruent condition. These components are commonly identified in the Stroop, the Simon, the Switch and the Flanker tasks.

The first conflict-related ERP component is N200. Studies indicate that incongruent conditions show an increase in the frontal negativity (N200) which might be related to the trade-off between inhibition and activation of the non-target and target lexical items. A long-lasting mid-frontal negative component might reflect the amount of cognitive control required to process a specific task in one language. In switching settings, this mid-frontal negative component is larger for the dominant than for the non-dominant language, and in comparison to monolinguals, bilinguals should show a larger mid-frontal negativity related to the degree of cognitive control required to process a specific language (Moreno et al., 2008).

By using ERP, we can compare wave forms (brain responses) of inhibitory condition to those of non-inhibitory condition. We usually examine the following indexes. One is a middle-right frontal N200 effect that is associated with response inhibition. Another is the difference waveforms that are computed by subtracting the GO condition from the no-GO condition (see Figure 13).

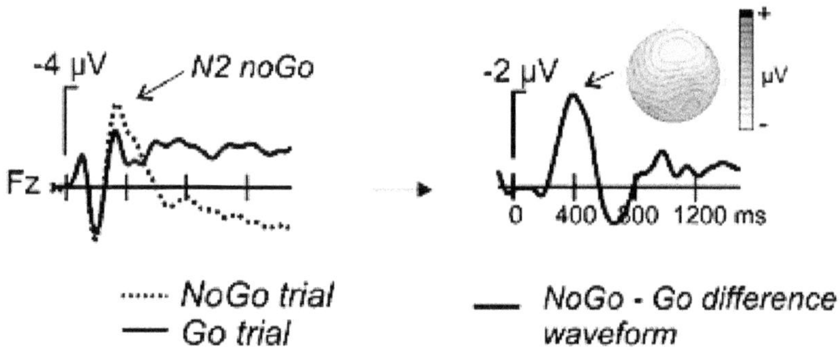

Figure 13. Wave forms of N2 effect and difference waveforms between GO and no-GO condition in GO/no-GO ERP paradigm (Rodriguez-Fornells, Rotte, Heinze, Nosselt, & Munte, 2002).

The second conflict-related ERP component is LPC (late positive component), which is referred to as slow positivity or slow potential sometimes. In the conflict resolution task such as the Stroop, the LPC is identified as positivity in the incongruent condition compared to the congruent or control conditions, occurring from approximately 600–900 ms post-stimulus (Appelbaum, Meyerhoff, & Woldorff, 2009).

Although the source of LPC remains unspecified, a few studies (West, 2003) tried to trace the LPC to the inferior frontal gyrus and left extrastriate region, and the results suggested that this component indicated conflict resolution processes. It was suggested that the amplitude of the LPC has been correlated with RT and accuracy, and the LPC reflects response selection (West, Jakubek, Wymbs, Perry, & Moore, 2005). In language switching paradigm, it was suggested that the LPC switching effect is indexing the reconfiguration of stimulus-response linkage to the previously suppressed lexicon. This positivity might correspond to a similar positive switching component isolated in other ERP studies and be related to task-set reconfiguration processes when processing cues indexing an incoming switch (Jackson, Swainson, Cunnington, & Jackson, 2001; Moreno et al., 2008). Despite the ambiguous underlying function of this component, the LPC is nevertheless reliably activated during conflict processing. In comparing the latency and amplitude of N200 and LPC components between monolinguals and bilinguals (or between different types of bilinguals), we are able to see the neurocognitive differences in cognitive control when they perform conflict-related tasks.

fMRI Measurement

The method of fMRI, which has sensitive and high space resolution, provides a unique way to study the loci of language processing in bilinguals' brain and allows us to see what neuro-structures are involved in language control. The fMRI data in GO/no-GO experiments showed that two regions are associated with the non-coincidence effect in bilinguals when compared to monolinguals (Rodriguez-Fornells et al., 2005): The left dorso-lateral prefrontal cortex (DLPFC) and the supplementary motor area (SMA). Interestingly, these areas are also associated with executive control of other tasks, suggesting that bilinguals use "typical" executive function brain areas (Rodriguez-Fornells et al., 2005). The roles of associated brain areas of the left DLPFC/ACC-SMA net-work have been suggested to include different aspects of cognitive control (Rodriguez-Fornells, Balaguer, & Munte, 2006), such as (a) the selection of different response alternatives (b) the switching between tasks (c) the maintenance of a stable representation of the current task and prevention of interference and (d) the inhibition of irrelevant items held in working memory.

Based on neuroimaging data, Abutalebi and Green (2007) concluded that the neural representation of a second language converges with the representation of that language learned as a first language and that language production in bilinguals is a dynamic process involving cortical and sub-cortical structures that make use of general cognitive control (e.g., inhibition) to resolve lexical competition and to select the intended language (Abutalebi & Green, 2007) (Figure 14). They proposed a neural network of multiple levels of *cognitive control* and bilingual language production, which comprehensively specifies the presumed functions of each brain area related to *language control* in bilingual language processing. Typically, Prefrontal Cortex (PFC) is mainly responsible for executive functions such as decision-making, response selection, inhibition, and working memory, while Anterior Cingulate Cortex (ACC) is mainly responsible for attention, conflict monitoring, and error detection (Abutalebi & Green, 2008; Abutalebi et al., 2012; Luk, Green, Abutalebi, & Grady, 2012). In comparing the brain activations related to cognitive control, we are able to collect data that indicate qualitative differences of cognitive control mechanism between monolinguals and bilinguals, or between different types of bilinguals.

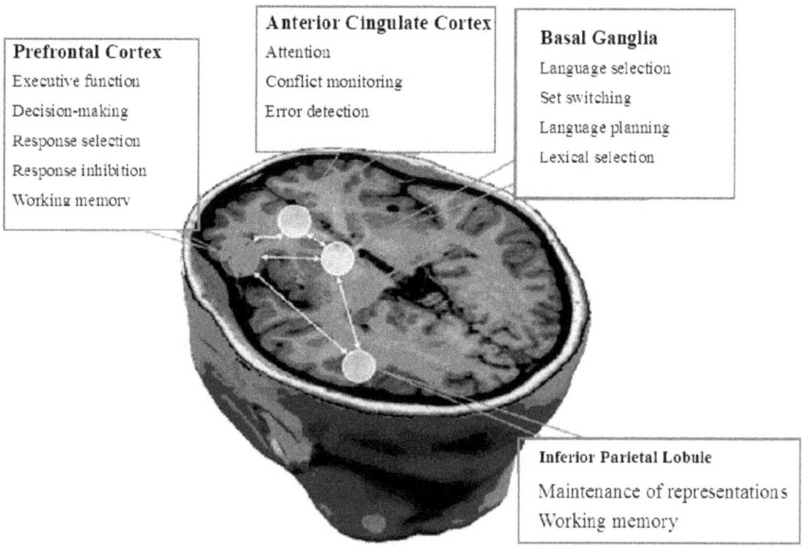

Figure 14. Multiple levels of cognitive control and bilingual language production (Abutalebi & Green, 2007).

2.3.2 Evidence of Bilingual Advantage

Bilingualism induces significant consequences on bilinguals' cognitive development. Bilingual advantage, in a narrow sense, refers to bilinguals' superior performance relative to monolinguals on tasks requiring cognitive control. As introduced above, the tasks that have been commonly used for measuring cognitive control include the Stroop task, the Simon task, the Flanker task, the Attention Network task, the Switch task, and the Card Sorting task (Bialystok et al., 2004; Bialystok, Martin, & Viswanathan, 2005; Carlson & Meltzoff, 2008; Costa et al., 2009; Marian, Blumenfeld, Mizrahi, Kania, & Cordes, 2013; Martin-Rhee & Bialystok, 2008). Combined with behavioral measurements, new techniques such as ERPs and fMRI have also been adopted in some studies.

Since the 1960s, a growing number of studies demonstrate that bilinguals show advantages in cognitive control, particularly in the aspects of inhibitory control (inhibition), conflict monitoring, and mental set shifting, as speaking two languages requires controlling one's attention, monitoring the use of the target language, inhibiting irrelevant information, and switching between different languages (Bialystok et al., 2009; Christoffels, Kroll, & Bajo, 2013; Kroll & Bialystok, 2013; Peal & Lambert, 1962). Now I will review the literature according to different age groups: *child bilinguals, mid-age and older adult bilinguals, and young adult bilinguals.*

2.3.2.1 Child Bilinguals

Early studies on bilingual advantage started from the comparisons between child bilinguals and their counterpart monolinguals in performing some cognitive control tasks. In one of the early studies (Bialystok, 1986), monolingual and bilingual children between 5 and 9 year old were asked to complete a *grammaticality judgment task*, in which children were required to judge whether the sentence presented was grammatical or not, even when the sentence was semantically meaningless (e.g. Apples grow on noses), and a *sentence grammar correction task*, in which children were required to correct grammatical errors of sentences. The results of this study showed that bilinguals demonstrated a superior performance in judgment task, which was consistent with expectation because bilinguals might have richer knowledge of languages. But more importantly, bilinguals also demonstrated higher control in *grammar correction task* because the task was assumed to deal with control processes since correcting the grammatical error required effort to control and inhibit sentence anomaly. The bilingual advantages were observed also in non-verbal tasks (Bialystok, 1987). The *dimensional change card sort task* was adopted (Bialystok, 1999) to tap executive control, which specifically required participants to sort cards on different dimensions, reflecting the ability to inhibit the more salient alternative and to change flexibly with the new rule. The results turned out that bilingual children showed significantly more correct responses than monolinguals. In a later study using the same task paradigm (Bialystok & Martin, 2004), 67 bilingual and monolingual children (58.9 months) participants were asked to complete the task with difficult representational demands. The results again showed that bilinguals have better inhibitory control for ignoring perceptual information than monolinguals do. In a study in the following year, it was replicated that bilingual children (5 years) were better, relative to their monolingual counterparts, at ignoring misleading information by conducting a *Simon task* (Bialystok et al., 2005). A more recent study (Martin-Rhee & Bialystok, 2008) further demonstrated that bilingual advantages were more obvious in complex tasks requiring control over attention to competing cues (interference suppressions). In the research, Study 1 replicated previous findings that bilinguals were faster in performing the Simon task compared to monolinguals, but only in high demand condition of inhibitory control. Study 2 and Study 3 showed that bilingual children maintained better performance on task requiring control of attention but not on task underlying response inhibition. Bilingual advantages were observed also in bilingual children from different cultures, thus further proving the generality of bilingual advantage (Bialystok & Viswanathan, 2009). In the study, 90 children (8 years) from three groups (monolinguals in Canada, bilinguals in Canada, and bilinguals in India) were required to complete a behavioral version of an *anti-saccade task* – faces task – to isolate 3 different components (response suppression, inhibitory control, and cognitive flexibility) of executive control. The results indicated that the bilingual children from both cultures were faster than monolinguals on inhibitory control and cognitive flexibility but there was no difference between groups on response suppression or on a control condition involving no executive control. Furthermore, there was no group difference between the two bilinguals, but both bilingual groups were significantly better than the monolinguals on all measures. In a study by adopting *Global-Local and Trail-Making Tasks* (Bialystok, 2010), the performances of 151 bilingual and monolingual children (6 years) were compared. The results demonstrated that there was bilingual advantage in processing complex stimuli in tasks requiring switching and updating, even when no inhibition involved. In other recent studies (Feng, Bialystok, & Diamond, 2009; Morales, Calvo, & Bialystok, 2013; Soliman, 2014), it was reported that bilingual children also show advantage in working memory. In their studies, bilingual children performed significantly better than monolinguals when they were executing tasks requiring high demands of working memory. In addition, it was reported that bilingual training extends their working memory span, thus enabling bilinguals to control more efficiently in a highly intensive context (Tzou, Eslami, Chen, & Vaid, 2011; Weldon, Mushlin, Kim, & Sohn, 2013).

The studies reviewed above reveal that bilingual children enjoy more advantages in different aspects of cognitive control such as inhibition, switching, and working memory. For child bilinguals, the learning of two languages usually takes place simultaneously, so they are more often balanced bilinguals or sometimes called early bilinguals. In previous studies it is suggested that bilingual advantage is independent of language difference, cultural background, and language of schooling (e.g., Barac & Bialystok, 2012), and it is also suggested that bilingual advantage is more sensitive to detection among child bilinguals as compared with bilinguals in other age groups. Next, I will review bilingual advantage among the mid-age and older adult bilinguals.

2.3.2.2 Mid-age and Older Adult Bilinguals

The bilingual advantage extends to mid-age and older adult bilinguals. One early study of such kind attempted to find out whether the bilingual advantage of cognitive control persists for mid-age adults and for older adult bilinguals (Bialystok et al., 2004). In the study, mid-age and older adult bilinguals and counterpart monolinguals were required to complete the *Simon task*. There were three sub-studies. Study 1 was to investigate the possible effects of adult aging and language group by the Simon task. There were 40 participants who were classified into two age groups: one of mid-age group (43.0 years), the other of older age group (71.9 years). Each group was composed of half monolinguals and half bilinguals. The results showed that the bilinguals were consistently faster in responding to the Simon task and showed smaller Simon effect compared to the monolinguals. In addition, the older bilinguals also showed fewer errors than the older monolinguals. Study 2, based on the preliminary results of Study 1, was to replicate the patterns of age and language group and to isolate the source of bilingual advantage by including two conditions in which working memory demands were increased to determine whether this manipulation also favored bilinguals. The first age group consisted of 64 participants (42.6 years), half monolinguals and half bilinguals. The second age group consisted of 30 participants (70.3 years), half monolinguals and half bilinguals. Similarly, each group was required to complete the Simon task; only the Simon task varied in working memory demand by 4 varying conditions. The results of Study 2 showed firstly a smaller Simon effect for the bilinguals, secondly a reduction of age-related processing costs, and thirdly a reliable attenuation of age-related Simon effect and work memory costs. Study 3 was to determine whether the two language groups (10 monolinguals with 38.8 years, 10 bilinguals with 40.6 years) would eventually converge in their performance after sufficient practice. Results showed that the two groups differed in their performance of the Simon task, but the performance of the two groups converged eventually, reflecting great practice effect. The results of the three studies revealed that bilinguals performed better than monolinguals on the Simon task both in overall RTs and in the Simon effect. And the advantage was greater for the older participants. Bialystok et al. suggested that bilingualism might help to off-set age-related losses in executive control.

In a later study (Bialystok et al., 2007), the effect of lifelong bilingualism on maintaining cognitive functioning was examined. 184 patients diagnosed with dementia were examined, of whom 51% were bilinguals. The results demonstrated that bilinguals showed symptoms of *dementia* four years later than monolinguals, suggesting that bilingualism might delay the onset of symptoms of dementia in old age. In another study (Bialystok et al., 2008), ninety-six younger (20 years) or older (68 years) adults and either monolinguals or bilinguals were compared when they performed tasks assessing working memory, lexical retrieval, and executive control. The results indicated that there was similar performance between monolinguals and bilinguals on working memory tasks, monolinguals were significantly better than bilinguals on lexical retrieval tasks, but bilinguals were superior to monolinguals on executive tasks. More importantly, evidence showed that there were larger language group differences in older participants on the executive control tasks. These results revealed that the beneficial effect of bilingualism on cognitive control persists to older adulthood and remains even larger for aged-groups of bilinguals relative to younger bilinguals.

Studies show that bilingualism also contributes to *cognitive reserve,* which acts to compensate for cognitive dysfunction, damaging or aging. In this way, it was suggested lifelong bilingualism confers protection against the onset of Alzheimer disease (AD) (Bialystok et al., 2007; Craik, Bialystok, & Freedman, 2010). In Craik et al. (2010)'s study, 102 bilingual AD patients and 109 monolingual AD patients were compared. With the matching of other confounding factors such as education, occupational status, or immigration, the results showed that the bilingual patients had been diagnosed 4.3 years later and had reported the onset of symptoms 5.1 years later than the monolingual counterparts (Craik et al., 2010).

A more recent study provides direct evidence of *a neural basis* for the bilingual cognitive control boost in aging (Gold, Kim, Johnson, Kryscio, & Smith, 2013). 110 subjects of younger and older monolinguals and bilinguals participated in the perceptual switching task experiments. In experiment 1, older adult bilinguals (64.1 years) showed better perceptual switching performance than their monolingual counterparts (63.3 years). In experiment 2, younger (32.2 years) monolinguals and bilinguals (31.6 years) and older monolinguals and bilinguals completed the same switching task and at the same time fMRI was recorded. The results showed that bilingual older adults outperformed monolinguals and displayed decreased activation in left lateral frontal cortex and cingulate cortex. Importantly, this decreased activation associated with bilingualism was directly correlated with better task-switching performance.

From what has been presented, it can be inferred that the beneficial effect of bilingualism is prevalent among the mid-age and older adult bilinguals compared with their monolingual peers. Particularly, for older adult bilinguals, this effect is more significant in that bilingualism contributes to cognitive reserve, which helps bilinguals to stay in normal cognitive control functioning, thus delaying the onset of dementia (Schweizer, Ware, Fischer, Craik, & Bialystok, 2012).

2.3.2.3 Young Adult Bilinguals

Finally, I will present a review of bilingual advantage in cognitive control among young adult bilinguals. The research results of young adult bilinguals demonstrate a mixed picture.

The beneficial effect of bilingualism among young adult bilinguals was not as obvious as in child bilinguals and older adult bilinguals. In one such study, different age levels of bilingual and monolingual groups were compared (Bialystok et al., 2005). The groups were classified into 5-year-olds, young, middle-aged, and older adults performing the same task, the *Simon task.* These comparative studies demonstrated a substantial bilingual advantage (faster RTs) in the 5-year-old children, virtually absent in 20-year-old undergraduate participants, but present again in groups of middle-aged (30–59) and older (60–80) adults. In another study attempting to examine the effect of bilingualism and aging on executive control (Bialystok et al., 2006), two studies were conducted. In Study 1, one group was 24 young monolinguals (20.7 years) and 24 young bilinguals (20.8 years); the other group was 24 older monolinguals (70.4 years) and 24 older bilinguals (71.3 years). All the participants were required to complete a modified *anti-saccade task.* The results showed no group difference either in global RTs or in executive control index. In Study 2, there were 24 young bilinguals (23.9 years) and monolinguals (25.6 years) respectively, and 24 older bilinguals (64.5 years) and monolinguals (66.9 years) respectively. The study replicated results similar to Study 1: differences were observed only between older bilinguals and monolingual groups; there was no difference between young bilinguals and young monolinguals in performing the task. It was suggested that the absence of bilingual advantage for young bilinguals may reflect the fact that cognitive control is at the peak of efficiency at that time, so bilingualism provides no further boost (Bialystok et al., 2009; Bialystok et al., 2005). Similarly, particularly in behavioral measures, there have been quite a few studies that did not capture positive results of bilingual advantages among young adult bilinguals (e.g., Colzato et al., 2008; Costa et al., 2009; Kousaie & Phillips, 2012a; Luk et al., 2010; Paap & Greenberg, 2013).

However, there are also behavioral studies that support bilingual advantage among young adult bilinguals. In order to explore the effect of bilingualism on attentional networks, a study was conducted by comparing monolinguals and bilinguals in the *Attentional Network Task* (Costa, Hernandez, & Sebastian-Galles, 2008). 100 Catalan-Spanish early bilinguals (22 years) and 100 Spanish monolinguals (22 years) participated in the study. Language proficiency was matched and the bilinguals were balanced. The Attentional Network Task (ANT) was assumed to examine three different attentional networks: alerting, orienting and executive control. The results showed that bilinguals performed better than monolinguals in the task: bilinguals were more efficient in the alerting and executive control networks, revealing better ability of resolving conflict information. In addition, after analyzing switch costs between different trial types, it suggested that bilinguals had a smaller switch costs than monolinguals. These results proved that bilingualism exerts a positive effect on attentional control among young adult bilinguals, who are said to be at the peak of their cognitive control efficiency. In a later study (Costa et al., 2009), two experiments were conducted to explore in detail the bilingual advantage in conflict resolution task by adopting the *Flanker task*. But the Flanker task was designed in two versions, one in low-monitoring demand, and the other in high-monitoring demand. The Flanker type included congruent and incongruent trials. A total of 244 undergraduate students participated in the two experiments. In low-monitoring version of the Flanker task where most of the trials were just one type, the results demonstrated that there was no group difference in overall reaction times. However, in high-monitoring version of the Flanker task where most of the trials were evenly distributed, the results showed bilinguals were significantly faster in overall reaction times, revealing that bilinguals were better at recruiting a good deal of monitoring resources. To provide new evidence regarding the impact of bilingualism on attentional control, Hernandez et al. (2010) adopted a *numerical Stroop task* to investigate the issue. 54 young bilinguals (20.55 years) and monolinguals (21.15 years) were compared to assess the executive control network in Experiment 1. The experiment result showed more efficient performance for the bilingual group. Experiment 2 was modified by adding visual cue to assess the orienting network. The experiment demonstrated similar result, indicating the positive effect of bilingualism on cognitive control (Hernandez, Costa, Fuentes, Vivas, & Sebastian-Galles, 2010). Some more recent studies used *task-switching paradigm* to investigate whether young bilinguals would be more efficient in mental flexibility compared to counterpart monolinguals (Prior & Gollan, 2011; Prior & Macwhinney, 2010). In Prior and Macwhinney's study (2010), the performance of monolinguals and fluent bilingual college students were compared by requiring participants to complete a task switch. Task-switching paradigm was supposed to tap the ability to shift between mental sets. The results demonstrated that there was no group difference in mix costs (difference between repetition trials of mix block and trials of single block) but there was significant reduced switch costs (difference between non-switch trials and switch trials in mix block) for the young adult bilinguals. A later study by Prior and Gollan (2011) replicated these results and further suggested that bilinguals with more frequent language switching practices performed better than bilinguals with less language switching practices, revealing an explicit link between language-switching and bilingual advantages in task-switching. In some studies measuring mental set shifting, it was further found that bilingualism has a significant role in bilinguals' enhancement of cognitive control, by using another sort of experiment paradigm, *Card Sorting Change task.* For example, in a study of this kind, it was proved that bilinguals like professional interpreters are significantly better at mental set shifting than control bilinguals and monolinguals or compared to the time before interpreting training (Festman & Munte, 2012; Macnamara & Conway, 2014; Yudes et al., 2011).

Furthermore, given the absence of a bilingual advantage among young adults in behavioral measurement, electrophysiological studies were conducted by adopting MEG, ERPs or fMRI techniques to determine the neural correlates of the bilingual advantage previously reported for behavioral measures in conflict tasks. One study (Bialystok et al., 2005) used magneto-encephalography (MEG) to examine whether the brain responses would be different between young adult bilinguals and counterpart monolinguals when they perform the Simon task. There were three groups in the study, one group of monolinguals and two groups of bilinguals (Cantonese-English and French-English). The results showed that the French-English bilinguals and monolinguals presented similar performance in behavioral measures (overall speed), but the imaging data showed difference between the two bilingual groups and the monolingual group. Specifically, there was greater activation in the right temporal and left frontal and cingulate areas for the bilinguals, which was associated with faster responding in the bilinguals. ERPs studies have shown that bilinguals exert higher cognitive control than monolinguals (Morales, Yudes, Gomez-Ariza, & Bajo, 2015; Moreno, Wodniecka, Tays, Alain, & Bialystok, 2014; Sullivan, Janus, Moreno, Astheimer, & Bialystok, 2014). For example, Fernandez, Tartar, Padron, and Acosta (2013) compared English monolinguals to Spanish-English bilinguals on event related potentials (ERPs) by adopting a nonlinguistic auditory Go/noGo Task which tested inhibitory control. It was found that bilinguals showed greater mean N2 amplitude (inhibition) than monolinguals, but both groups performed the task equally well. This finding has provided the link between bilingual advantage and a neural correlate of inhibition(Fernandez, Tartar, Padron, & Acosta, 2013). In neuroimaging studies (fMRI), similarly, it has been reported that bilingualism greatly tunes brain network and mechanism associated with cognitive control. Compared to monolinguals, bilinguals have stronger brain activation in related areas (dorsal precentral gyrus, pars triangularis, pars opercularis, superior temporal gyrus, and planum temporale), possibly as a result of simultaneous activation of two languages and competitive selection of target language in language production, which involves the participation of cognitive control to avoid inter-language interference (Abutalebi, 2008; Abutalebi et al., 2012; Parker et al., 2012).

Therefore, it can be assumed that even when there is no difference between bilinguals and monolinguals on cognitive control in behavioral measures it is still possible that the underlying neural processes may be different between monolingual and bilingual groups (Kousaie, 2011).

2.3.2.4 Summary of the Literature

The studies of bilingual advantage in cognitive control are numerous. Positive evidence of bilingual advantage has been found in various bilinguals, particularly in children and old adults. However, it should be noted that a few recent studies do not support the existence of bilingual advantage, particularly among young adult bilinguals (e.g., Anton et al., 2014; Gathercole et al., 2014; Kirk, Fiala, Scott-Brown, & Kempe, 2014; Kousaie, Sheppard, Lemieux, Monetta, & Taler, 2014; Paap & Greenberg, 2013), even though the evidence of bilingual advantage among child bilinguals and mid-age/older age bilinguals is not absolutely positive (e.g., Gathercole et al., 2014). Therefore, the lack or inconsistence of evidence suggests that bilingual advantage should be further scrutinized especially in terms of which bilinguals, if any, enjoy bilingual advantage, and under what conditions and why.

To conclude, the idea that bilingualism leads to cognitive control enhancement (bilingual advantage) is widely accepted. Hypothetically, null evidence in a few studies does not deny the existence of bilingual advantage. It is logical that advantage in cognitive control may not be detected in some groups of bilinguals because of variations of measurement, changes of context, degrees of bilingualism, and differences of bilingual experiences.

2.3.3 Relevant Factors Affecting Cognitive Control

Besides bilingualism, there are a few other factors that are closely related to cognitive control and may modulate individuals' cognitive control abilities in one way or another. In the following paragraphs, I include age, intelligence, and social economic status (SES) as the most influential ones.

Age

Cognitive control abilities mature at different rates over time. Some abilities mature in late childhood whereas others in early adulthood. As time goes by, cognitive control abilities decline gradually. Some abilities decline earlier, whereas others decline until older age (70, for example).

During the processes of developing, maturing, and declining, cognitive control abilities can be shaped by both physical changes in the brain and by life experiences. Cognitive control development is reported to be associated with the neuro-physiological development of the brain. Studies observe that when the processing capacity of related brain regions (such as the frontal lobes and other connected regions) increases, the core cognitive control functions also emerge (Anderson, 2002; De Luca & Leventer, 2008). Once the functions are established, they continue to mature. Some complex functions grow and develop for a long time, whereas others may mature in spurts. For example, some basic cognitive control abilities such as inhibitory control and working memory appear earliest with initial signs observed in 7–12-month old infants. Later on, based on inhibitory control and working memory, it is possible for more complex cognitive functions such as problem-solving to develop (Senn, Espy, & Kaufmann, 2004). Preschool children between the age of 3 to 5 years may have a boom in inhibition and working memory development (Best, Miller, & Jones, 2009). Also during this time, cognitive flexibility, goal-directed behavior, and planning begin to develop. However, they do not have fully mature executive functions and continue to make errors related to these emerging abilities. The fact is that they already have these abilities, but they make errors probably because they do not know how and when to use these particular strategies in specific contexts. In preadolescent time, some abilities continue to grow gradually and others may spurt, which indicates that the cognitive control development does not necessarily occur in a linear manner. During this period, children may display major increases in verbal working memory (Brocki & Bohlin, 2004), goal-directed behavior (with a potential spurt around 12 years of age) (Anderson, Anderson, Northan, Jacobs, & Catroppa, 2001), response inhibition and selective attention (Klimkeit, Mattingley, Sheppard,

Farrow, & Bradshaw, 2004), and strategic planning and organizational skills. Additionally, between the ages of 8 to 10, cognitive flexibility in particular begins to match adult levels (De Luca et al., 2003; Luciana & Nelson, 2002). However, similar to patterns in childhood development, executive functioning in preadolescents is limited because they do not reliably apply these executive functions across multiple contexts as a result of ongoing development of inhibitory control. Many executive functions may begin in childhood and preadolescence, such as inhibitory control. Yet, it is during adolescence when the different brain systems become better integrated. At this time, the adolescents execute cognitive control functions such as inhibitory control more efficiently and effectively, and cognitive control will improve throughout this time period (Leon-Carrion, García-Orza, & Pérez-Santamaría, 2004; Luna, Garver, Urban, Lazar, & Sweeney, 2004). Just as inhibitory control emerges in childhood and improves over time, planning and goal-directed behavior also demonstrate an extended time course with ongoing growth over adolescence (Anderson et al., 2001; Best et al., 2009). Likewise, functions such as attentional control, with a potential spurt at age 15 (Anderson et al., 2001), along with working memory (Luna et al., 2004), continue developing at this stage.

The major change that occurs in the brain in adulthood is the constant myelination of neurons in the prefrontal cortex. At age 20–29, executive functioning skills are at their peak, which allows people of this age to participate in some of the most challenging mental tasks. These skills begin to decline in later adulthood. Working memory and spatial span are areas where decline is most readily noted. Cognitive flexibility, however, has a late onset of impairment and does not usually start declining until around age 70 in normally functioning adults (De Luca & Leventer, 2008). Impaired executive functioning has been found to be the best predictor of functional decline in the elderly.

In the studies of bilingual advantage in cognitive control, a large amount of studies show that bilingual advantages are greater for child and older bilinguals than for young adult bilinguals. It appears, therefore, that controlled processing is carried out more effectively by bilinguals and that bilingualism helps to facilitate cognitive functions and offset age-related losses in certain executive processes (Bialystok et al., 2004; Bialystok et al., 2007; Gold et al., 2013). The absence of an advantage in young adult bilinguals may come from the fact that cognitive control is most efficient at that time, so bilingualism provides no further boost (Bialystok et al., 2009; Bialystok et al., 2005). Therefore, in investigating bilingual advantage, age is an important factor that needs to be strictly controlled. Child bilinguals (usually children whose cognitive control is still under development), young adult bilinguals (20–29), mid-age bilinguals (usually 40s–50s), and older adult bilinguals (60s–) are usually distinguished.

Intelligence
Accumulating evidence suggests that cognitive control abilities are related to intelligence, despite neuro-psychological results initially considered evidence of no such relation (Friedman et al., 2006) in some aspects. Intelligence, as measured on many commonly used tests, is often separated into verbal and nonverbal scores, which can be combined to produce a full-scale intelligence score. There are two categories: fluid intelligence and crystallized intelligence. Fluid intelligence means the reasoning abilities that can work across different domains such as in a novel task. Usually it can be measured by tasks requiring abstract reasoning such as figural analogies, Raven Matrices, and series completion. Crystallized intelligence refers to the declarative knowledge acquired from acculturated learning experiences. It is often measured by tasks such as vocabulary test, verbal comprehension, and general knowledge measures. In addition, there are other things like memory and learning, auditory perception, and processing speed. More importantly, all of these components are correlated with each other and with the general factor (Toplak, Sorge, Benoit, West, & Stanovich, 2010).

Most of the previous studies concerning bilingual advantage controlled the factor of intelligence. For this purpose, participants were required to complete an IQ test. The most commonly used tests (Toplak et al., 2010) are Matrices subtest-Kaufman brief intelligence test (Prior & Gollan, 2011), the Wechsler measures of intelligence, the Stanford Binet, Raven's Progressive Matrices, the Shipley Institute of Living Scale (Barry & Petry, 2008), PPVT (Bialystok et al., 2010), Verbal Fluency (Bialystok et al., 2009), and measures of intelligence from other languages (such as the German version of the WAIS) (Losel & Schmucker, 2004).

However, the finding that cognitive control is not unitary raises the issue of how intelligence relates to different aspects of cognitive control. In a study conducted by Friedman et al. (2006), the relations of fluid and crystallized intelligence and Wechsler Adult Intelligence Scale IQ to three separable components of cognitive control – inhibiting prepotent responses (inhibiting), shifting mental sets (shifting), and updating working memory (updating) – in young adults were examined. The results found that updating was highly correlated with the intelligence measures, but inhibiting and shifting were not. The results indicate that intelligence measures differentially relate to these three cognitive control aspects, suggesting that current intelligence measures do not equally assess a wide range of cognitive control abilities (Friedman et al., 2006).

Social Economic Status

Socioeconomic status (SES) is an economic and sociological measure of a person's work experience and of an individual's or family's economic and social position in relation to others, based on income, education, and occupation. When analyzing a family's SES, the household income, earners' education, and occupation are examined, as well as combined income, versus with an individual, when their own attributes are assessed. Socioeconomic status (SES) is strongly associated with cognitive ability and achievement during childhood and beyond. Little is known about the developmental relationships between SES and specific brain systems or their associated cognitive functions (Noble, Norman, & Farah, 2005). SES is reported to be an important predictor of neurocognitive performance, particularly of language and executive function, and that SES differences are found in neural processing even when performance levels are equal (Hackman & Farah, 2009). Current knowledge of socioeconomic status and child development indicates that children from higher-socioeconomic status families display better executive function – the ability to actively direct, control and regulate thoughts and behavior – than children from low-socioeconomic status families (Hook, Lawson, & Farah, 2013). In a recent study (Prior & Gollan, 2011), bilingual advantage was observed on switch cost only when SES was matched between groups. In another earlier study (Carlson & Meltzoff, 2008), a similar conclusion was reached when comparing English speaking monolinguals and Spanish-English bilingual pre-school children; despite an SES disadvantage for the bilinguals, the two groups performed similarly on tasks of executive function. These results displayed that SES might be an important variable that influence cognitive control.

However, the SES effect might be more influential in childhood bilinguals rather than adulthood bilinguals when other conditions are similar, because childhood bilinguals do not have a completely matured cognitive control system whereas adulthood bilinguals are already in the peak of cognitive control functions. In addition, the existence of socioeconomic status-related differences in executive function and brain function does not in any way imply that these differences are innate or unchangeable. The brain is a highly plastic organ; in fact, an emerging body of research demonstrates that the neural correlates of cognition can be changed by environmental experience (Rosenzweig, 2003).

Age, intelligence, and SES are three crucial factors modulating cognitive control in varied ways. Most previous studies have included age, intelligence, and SES as controlling variables for the study of bilingual advantage. There are usually two ways for doing this. First, we may keep these factors as constants. Second, we may resort to statistical methods to control them.

2.4 Summary

This chapter has presented a general review of the current research regarding bilingual advantage. The main points are summarized as below.

Firstly, in the language processing mechanism for bilinguals, both the two languages are activated simultaneously and non-selectively.

Secondly, bilinguals adopt some language control mechanisms to manage their two activated languages in order to avoid interference and intrusion from the non-target language when the target language is used.

Thirdly, the similarities between bilingual language control and general cognitive control suggest the existence of bilingual advantage in cognitive control.

Fourthly, the studies selected present a general review in support of bilingual advantage; however, a few studies do suggest that there is no significant difference between matched bilinguals and monolinguals in cognitive control tasks particularly among young adult bilinguals.

Chapter 3: Research Rationale and Questions

The previous chapter has presented the findings and the methods of previous research in the area of bilingual advantage. This chapter will, generally rather than specifically, present the current research rationale and research questions. More systematic and specific research background will be presented for each research question in their respective sections. Finally, some general hypotheses in response to the proposed questions will be formulated and four corresponding experiments will be laid out in general outline.

3.1 Research Rationale

As reviewed in the previous chapter, the topic of bilingual advantage has received a great deal of attention in the recent scientific and popular literature. Since the first positive evidence found in the 1960s (Peal & Lambert, 1962), numerous studies reveal that bilinguals perform more efficiently on tasks requiring cognitive control relative to monolinguals. Generally speaking, consistent evidence mainly comes from comparisons of cognitive control differences in the performance of cognitive control tasks between child bilinguals, older adult bilinguals and their counterpart monolinguals.

However, among young adult bilinguals in behavioral measures, quite a few studies do not present consistent evidence in support of the existence of bilingual advantage, (Bialystok et al., 2008; Bialystok et al., 2005; Kousaie & Phillips, 2012a; Luk et al., 2010; Paap & Greenberg, 2013). In Paap and Greenberg (2013)'s research, for example, three studies were conducted to compare young bilinguals and monolinguals on 15 indicators of cognitive control by administering tasks including antisaccade, Simon, Flanker, and color-shape switching. The results show that there is no main effect of group for each of the measures. Similarly, an earlier study (Kousaie & Phillips, 2012b) does not find any behavioral differences between young bilinguals and monolinguals in the Stroop, Simon, or Flanker tasks. In another study, they again find no evidence of the existence of bilingual advantage in young or older adults and they suggest that bilingual advantage is limited in its effect (Kousaie & Phillips, 2012a). In another recent study (Gathercole et al., 2014), utilizing the tasks of Card Sorting, Simon, and metalinguistic judgment, bilingual advantage is not found either in simultaneous bilinguals or in sequential bilinguals, including young adult bilinguals. Therefore, incoherence still exists regarding bilingual advantage in cognitive control (Paap & Greenberg, 2013), particularly among young adult bilinguals.

Different factors may contribute to this incoherence. Cognitive control is related to several factors in varied ways. As already mentioned in the literature review, numerous studies show that compared to young adult bilinguals, early bilinguals and mid-age and old-age bilinguals are more likely to have enhanced cognitive control abilities (Bialystok et al., 2007; Bialystok et al., 2005; Schweizer et al., 2012; Schweizer et al., 2013). These results indicate that bilinguals' age is a very important factor modulating bilingual advantage in cognitive control (Bialystok et al., 2009; Salvatierra & Rosselli, 2011; Tao, Marzecova, Taft, Asanowicz, & Wodniecka, 2011). In addition, variables such as SES and IQ (Bialystok et al., 2009) may significantly affect cognitive control, as well as individual differences (Festman, Rodriguez-Fornells, & Munte, 2010), cultural difference (Bialystok & Viswanathan, 2009), and language similarity (van Heuven, Conklin, Coderre, Guo, & Dijkstra, 2011).

However, emphasizing external modulating variables rather than those relating to bilingualism itself is misleading and does not fundamentally solve critical questions relating to bilingual advantage. The study of bilingual advantage invites us to consider two core concepts, concepts which in previous research have not been adequately resolved. The first is the nature of bilingualism, i.e., what does it mean to be bilingual? The second is the nature of cognitive control, i.e., what is the construct of cognitive control? With a proper understanding of these two concepts, we may address the problem of incoherence in findings related to bilingual advantage.

Firstly, bilingual experiences are heterogeneous for different bilingual populations and groups. For example, some bilinguals speak L2 more often, some bilinguals listen to L2 more often, and others may only read or write in L2 more often. Different types of bilingual experiences may influence the development of cognitive control in different ways (Kaushanskaya & Prior, 2014). The bilingual participants who speak a variety of language pairs vary in degrees of bilingualism. These bilinguals differ in many ways, such as in how proficient they are in their two languages, how they use the two languages, and how frequently they code-switch or mix the two languages etc. (Prior & Gollan, 2011). Such variety of bilingual experience makes it very likely that bilingual advantage in cognitive control is manifested in different ways among different groups of bilinguals. As put by Valian (2014), the question is: what kinds of experiences will improve executive function (cognitive control)? The inconsistency in the findings of bilingual advantage may be largely due to the fact that individuals vary in the number and kinds of experiences they have that promote superior executive function (cognitive control) (Valian, 2014). Most previous studies do not distinguish different bilingual experiences and only generally compare bilinguals with monolinguals, so they do not allow a design to directly compare different bilingual groups, or an investigation of the extent to which one must be bilingual before exhibiting any advantage. Therefore, it is difficult to identify precisely what about bilingualism is critical for each observed effect (Prior & Gollan, 2011). Most previous studies rated participants' language learning background (history, education, language balance etc.) but did not characterize the patterns of how bilinguals use their languages. According to Green (2011), bilingual language control ability is closely related to the behavioral ecology of bilingual speakers, signifying the community context in which bilingual speakers typically use their two languages. Therefore, it is very likely that different bilingual experiences in behavioral ecology, which play a very important role in discriminating different bilingual groups, contribute significantly and distinctively to cognitive control differences in bilinguals. For example, some studies discuss the idea that language switching experience is closely associated with task switching in cognitive control (Hervais-Adelman, Moser-Mercer, & Golestani, 2011; Rodriguez-Fornells, Kramer, Lorenzo-Seva, Festman, & Munte, 2011; Soveri, Rodriguez-Fornells, & Laine, 2011). Two or three recent studies directly investigate the link between interpreting experience and cognitive control (Morales, Padilla, Gomez-Ariza, & Bajo, 2015; Woumans, Ceuleers, Linden, Szmalec, & W., 2015; Yudes et al., 2011). The results reveal that interpreters outperform not only monolinguals but also control bilinguals. These findings support the existence of bilingual advantage and also indicate that different patterns of bilingual language-use modulate the nature and extent of cognitive control advantage among bilingual populations. Therefore, the specific characteristics and patterns of bilingual experience, which have been largely ignored in the field, may be crucial factors confounding the existence of bilingual advantage in cognitive control.

Secondly, the construct of cognitive control is unitary but can be separated into different subcomponents and these subcomponents can be measured by different tasks. As stated in the previous term definitions, cognitive control is a unitary construct but can be separated into different, independent aspects, such as conflict monitoring, inhibition, mental set shifting, and working memory updating etc. (Green & Abutalebi, 2013; Miyake et al., 2000), and these different aspects can be measured by different tasks. Therefore, theoretically, in order to reveal the impact of bilingual experience on cognitive control, all these different aspects should be measured by multiple tasks. However, most previous studies adopted only one single task in one single study or used different tasks across different bilingual populations (Paap & Greenberg, 2013), which is contradictory to the understanding that cognitive control is a complex set of cognitive processes, the components of which are sometimes minimally correlated with each other, depending on the task (Valian, 2014). In this case, a null effect in one particular task does not necessarily mean null effect in another task. The insufficient use of measuring tasks may be another important factor responsible for the incoherent findings of bilingual advantage in cognitive control.

Therefore, if the way in which bilinguals use their languages affects different aspects/components of cognitive control, a single composite measuring of cognitive control between monolinguals and bilinguals cannot specify exactly what type of bilingual experiences may have caused the enhancement of some specific aspect(s)/components of cognitive control. Without an understanding of how bilingual experiences might affect performance in cognitive control tasks in different ways, and without proper measuring tasks, it would be difficult to explain the inconsistent findings relating to bilingual advantage.

Therefore, in order to solve or even partially solve these problems, the following issues are to be resolved in the current research regarding bilingual advantage in cognitive control.

i) Specify the particular bilingual experiences among different bilingual groups that may lead to specific components or aspects of advantage in cognitive control. For this purpose, the current research operationally classifies bilinguals into different groups; those who have different levels of L2 proficiency and those who differ in language-use experiences in production. Both of these are crucial characteristics demonstrating the heterogeneity of bilingual experiences.
ii) Examine different components or aspects of bilingual advantage in cognitive control by adopting different tasks and by comparing different bilingual groups. As mentioned above, previous research mostly adopted only a single task or used different single tasks in different studies when comparing the cognitive control differences between monolinguals and bilinguals. This method does not adequately provide a full image of bilingual advantage and does not help to sort out which aspect of bilingualism causes cognitive control advantage. The current research will adopt different tasks that measure different aspects of cognitive control, including *inhibition, conflict monitoring, and mental set shifting,* across different groups of bilinguals. According to the literature review discussed in 2.3.1.1 of the previous chapter, there are some typical tasks that have been used consistently for cognitive control measurement. For the current research, therefore,

we will adopt three typical tasks to measure inhibition, conflict monitoring, and mental set shifting. They are the Flanker task, Number Stroop task, and the WCST. Both the Flanker task and the Number Stroop task (the two also differ in cognitive demand) are used to measure inhibition and conflict monitoring, whereas the WCST is used to measure mental set shifting (Detailed information about the tasks will be presented in next chapter – Experiment 1). This methodology is new because most previous studies adopted only one single task and examined only one aspect of cognitive control.

iii) Explore the relationships between some main components or aspects of cognitive control and some particular bilingual experiences. Previous research does not show how a particular bilingual experience is related to a particular aspect of cognitive control. As discussed earlier, it is very likely that different types of bilingual experience contribute significantly to bilingual advantage in one or more particular aspect(s) of cognitive control.

iv) Examine bilingual advantage *among young-adult bilinguals*. Compared to child bilinguals and old age bilinguals, bilingual advantage is more difficult to detect among young adult bilinguals, probably because young adult bilinguals are at the peak of cognitive development, thus leaving smaller space for cognitive control to improve. However, if bilingual advantage really exists, we can still find it even among young adult bilinguals as long as we could isolate the effect of specific language experiences bilinguals have acquired. Therefore, the detection of bilingual advantage among young-adult bilinguals, whose cognitive control functioning is at the highest level, would greatly confirm the efficacy of the proposed approach which gives due regard to bilingual experience and its complex impacts on cognitive control.

In short, as bilinguals have various characteristics in different bilingual experiences, and cognitive control is diversified in several different subcomponents, it is very likely that specific bilingual experiences bring about the enhancement of only one or more specific aspect(s) of cognitive control (e.g. inhibition rather than shifting). A precise examination of bilingual advantage thus shall consider the corresponding association between specific characteristics of bilingual experience and specific aspects of cognitive control. To my knowledge, this doctoral research is the first to do so in the field.

3.2 Research Questions

As discussed earlier, bilingual advantage is not consistently observed, particularly among young-adult bilinguals. Quite a few studies report null effect of bilingual advantage on cognitive control among young-adult bilinguals (Gathercole et al., 2014; Kirk et al., 2014; Kousaie & Phillips, 2012a; Paap & Greenberg, 2013). One typical explanation for this null effect is that bilingualism confers no further boom in young-adult bilinguals because they are at the peak of cognitive control efficiency (Bialystok et al., 2009; Bialystok et al., 2012). We admit that age is one of the important factors that affect bilingual advantage (particularly in child and older adult bilinguals), but it does not fundamentally eliminate the bilingual effect among young-adult bilinguals. Our concern is to find out why and how such null effect is caused. As stated in the rationale, the inconsistency of bilingual advantage may not come from young age (thus being efficient in cognitive control) but from the heterogeneity of bilingual experience and/or the diversity of cognitive control construct. There may be a more complicated and dynamic corresponding relationship between different bilingual experiences and different aspects of cognitive control. Therefore, **the *General Question*** for the current research is:

If bilingual advantage really exists, do different bilingual experiences affect different aspect(s) of cognitive control among young adult bilinguals?

Combining the heterogeneity of bilingual experience and the diversity of cognitive control together, we **hypothesize** that bilinguals may be better at cognitive control than monolinguals, and that specific bilingual experiences may be related to bilingual advantage in specific aspects of cognitive control.

If we can identify the relationship between specific bilingual experience and specific aspects of cognitive control among young-adult bilinguals, we would be able to understand the nature and sort out the specific source of bilingual advantage. In order to answer the general question, ***four specific research questions*** are to be answered.

Before we discuss whether differences in bilingual experiences cause differences in cognitive control, it is necessary to answer a prerequisite question ***(Research Question 1)*****:**

Do young adult bilinguals really have advantage in cognitive control when compared with monolinguals?

If the answer is yes, then we can go on to explore the relationship between specific bilingual experiences and specific aspects of bilingual advantage in cognitive control. Thus, the main purposes of the current research are firstly to verify the existence of bilingual advantage and secondly to further examine bilingual advantage by looking at the differences of bilingual experiences and their respective impacts upon different aspects of cognitive control. As stated in our rationale, the heterogeneity of bilingual experiences may bring about differences of bilingual advantage in cognitive control. Regarding the specificity of bilingual experience, three features are distinguished in the current research in order to identify their relationships with bilingual advantage in cognitive control, thus forming three specific research questions respectively.

The first perspective by which we operationally distinguish bilingual experience (as mentioned in our rationale), between different bilingual groups, is language proficiency. Language proficiency, which can be defined generally as the ability of an individual to comprehend and produce an acquired language, is an essential element of bilingualism. We cannot discuss the issue of bilingual advantage without investigating language proficiency because without a certain level of language proficiency, bilingualism does not exist. As learning time accumulates, language proficiency generally increases among bilinguals. Bilinguals vary significantly in language proficiency, particularly in L2 proficiency among young-adult bilinguals as they are in different stages of L2 learning while their L1 is already in full development. How may these different degrees of L2 proficiency affect cognitive control? Several recent studies suggest that language proficiency, particularly L2 proficiency, significantly modulates bilingual advantage in cognitive control (e.g., Barac & Bialystok, 2012; Singh & Mishra, 2012; 2013). Bilinguals with higher L2 proficiency may perform better than bilinguals with lower L2 proficiency in the Stroop task, the target detection task, or the attentional network task (Mishra, Hilchey, Singh, & Klein, 2012; Tse & Altarriba, 2012; Videsott, Della Rosa, Wiater, Franceschini, & Abutalebi, 2012). These studies mainly investigate the effect of language proficiency upon inhibitory control, but the effect upon other aspects of cognitive control still remains unknown. Therefore, a comparison of multiple aspects of cognitive control between bilingual groups (that differ in the degrees of L2 proficiency), rather than between monolinguals and bilinguals, is necessary for understanding the specific relationship between bilingualism and cognitive control. Therefore, the research question ***(Research Question 2*)** for this issue is:

Does second language (L2) proficiency contribute to cognitive control differences among young-adult bilinguals?

Besides L2 proficiency differences, bilinguals also vary greatly in how they use their two languages. Whether or not bilinguals have a homogeneous L2 proficiency, it is very likely that they use languages in very different ways, resulting in distinctive language-use experiences. Therefore, identifying the specific characteristics in language-use experience and tracking their respective relationships to cognitive control, would be necessary and significant to the research of bilingual advantage in cognitive control. In this volume, we operationally investigate two specific types of language-use experiences in production: *language interpreting experience* and *public speaking experience*, which are addressed respectively by two specific research questions.

The third research question examines cognitive control differences between young-adult bilinguals who have language interpreting experience and those who do not. Language interpreting requires bilingual speakers to intensively switch between two languages both in language comprehension and language production. Several recent studies reveal that interpreting experience affects cognitive control. Bilinguals who switch languages more often perform better than bilinguals who switch languages less often in task switch (Prior & Gollan, 2011), and professional interpreters perform better than control bilinguals in the Wisconsin Card Sorting Test (Yudes et al., 2011). These findings suggest the necessity of investigating the role of interpreting experience (or intentional language switching experience) in enhancing cognitive control. We will thus investigate whether and how interpreting experience can enhance different aspects of cognitive control. Therefore, the research question for this issue is **(*Research Question 3*):**

Does language interpreting experience contribute to cognitive control differences among young-adult bilinguals?

Similarly, next specific research question examines cognitive control differences between bilinguals who have public speaking experience and those who do not. Public speaking is another type of bilingual experience. Public speaking requires speakers to address a formal topic in front of an audience, usually in one of the two languages. This experience, particularly L2 public speaking experience, demands that one should focus on the target language, maintain the goal of his discourse and monitor its progress and demands that one should inhibit interruptions from emotional anxiety, stress, and stage fright. This special context may significantly affect cognitive control in specific ways. Although there are no direct studies investigating this issue yet, some relevant studies do show that, in public speaking, speakers are continuously using cognitive control to regulate emotion (e.g., fear, stress, or anxiety) (Schel & Crone, 2013). Moreover, neurocognitive data show that such regulation activates the common neural areas (ACC) for cognitive control (Mueller, 2011). Therefore, public speaking experience may very likely enhance cognitive control, but this effect may emerge only in some specific aspects that are closely related to such experience. The specific research question for this issue thus is **(*Research Question 4*)**:

Does public speaking experience contribute to cognitive control differences among young-adult bilinguals?

3.3 Research Hypotheses

In order to answer the general question: "*Do different bilingual experiences affect different aspects of cognitive control among young-adult bilinguals?*", the four specific research questions require answers.

Based on the literature review and our research rationale discussed above, we propose four **hypotheses** accordingly.

Hypothesis 1: Young adult bilinguals will outperform monolinguals in cognitive control.

Hypothesis 2: L2 proficiency will contribute significantly to cognitive control differences among young-adult bilinguals, but only in specific aspect(s).

Hypothesis 3: Interpreting experience will contribute significantly to cognitive control differences among young-adult bilinguals, but only in specific aspect(s).

Hypothesis 4: Public speaking experience will contribute significantly to cognitive control differences among young-adult bilinguals, but only in specific aspect(s).

3.4 Research Design

In order to answer these research questions, the current research requires four specific experiments respectively. Figure 15 is provided below for reference. Specific research background for each research question and detailed information about participants and methods will be described in their respective sections in the following chapters.

Experiments:
Experiment 1 intends to verify the existence of bilingual advantage among young adult bilinguals by comparing cognitive control differences between young adult bilinguals and counterpart monolinguals.

Experiment 2 examines the role of L2 proficiency in bilingual advantage among young-adult bilinguals by comparing cognitive control differences between two groups of young-adult bilinguals who differ in L2 proficiency.

Experiment 3 explores the role of language interpreting experience in enhancing cognitive control among young-adult bilinguals by comparing cognitive control differences across four groups who differ in L2 proficiency and interpreting experience.

Experiment 4 explores the role of public speaking experience in enhancing cognitive control among young-adult bilinguals by comparing cognitive control differences across four groups who differ in L2 proficiency and public speaking experience.

Measuring Tasks:
As already discussed in our rationale, the crucial methodological shortcoming in previous research is that only a single task is adopted in a single study or different tasks are used across different studies. As cognitive control has multiple components, only one single task does not measure/cover the diversified aspects of cognitive control. Furthermore, the results of a single task do not lend themselves to comparison across different groups. In order to solve these problems, we adopt multiple tasks to measure different aspects of cognitive control, and administer the same tasks across all the four different experiments. The three different tasks are the Flanker task, the Number Stroop task, and the Wisconsin Card Sorting Test. These tasks have been widely used in the literature for cognitive control measurement. Both the Flanker task and the Number Stroop task measure different aspects of cognitive control, among them the aspects of inhibition and conflict monitoring, and the WCST measures one of its typical aspect – mental set shifting. Detailed descriptions of the three tasks will be presented in Experiment 1.

Do different bilingual experiences affect cognitive control in different aspects?

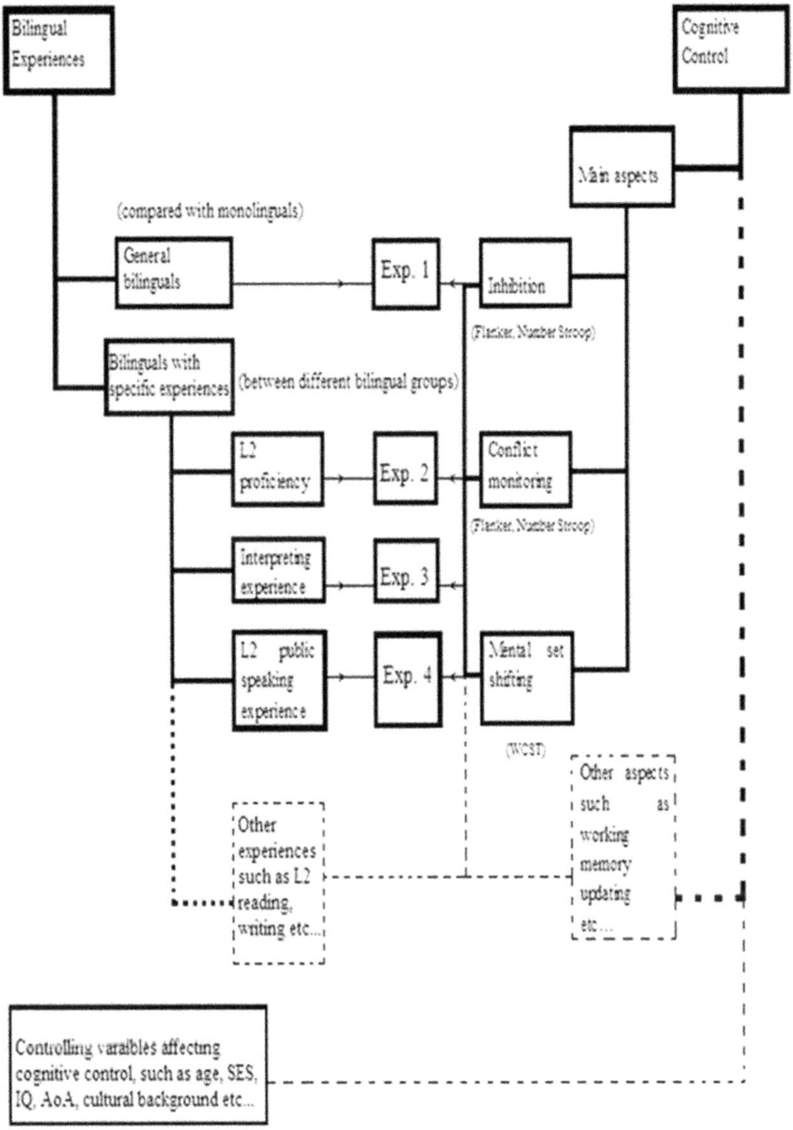

Figure 15. General outline of the current research.

3.5 Summary

This chapter discusses the research rationale and has posed research questions regarding the relationship between bilingual experience and cognitive control. General designs for the current research have been presented. The main points are summarized as followed.

Firstly, the research rationale discusses the existing problems regarding the heterogeneity of bilingual experience and the diversity of cognitive control, paving the way for the current research questions concerning bilingual advantage. These questions, including one general question and four specific questions, have been raised in order to solve the above-mentioned problems.

Secondly, theoretical hypotheses have been proposed corresponding with each of the four research questions.

Finally, a general design for the current research, which includes four specific experiments, has been presented. In the following chapters, I will examine the research questions individually along with their respective experiments.

Chapter 4: Experiment One – Bilingual Advantage in the Chinese Context

4.1 Introduction

In order to answer the general question "*Do different bilingual experiences affect cognitive control in different aspects among young adult bilinguals?*", a prerequisite question has to be answered. If the answer is yes, then we can go on to explore the relationship between specific bilingual experiences and specific aspects of bilingual advantage in cognitive control. The current experiment answers this prerequisite question – *Research Question 1* – by focusing on young adult bilinguals from the Chinese context: *Do young adult bilinguals have advantage in cognitive control compared to monolinguals?*

4.2 Specific Background

In most previous studies, bilingual participants were either Europeans or Americans or immigrants with heterogeneous L1 and culture background (Bialystok et al., 2010; Bialystok et al., 2005; Magezi, Khateb, Mouthon, Spierer, & Annoni, 2012; Paap & Greenberg, 2013). Few have ever directly examined bilinguals from homogeneous L1 and cultural background. For example, in Bialystok et al. (2010), the two monolingual groups were comprised of 37 French-speaking children in France, or 69 English-speaking children in Canada; whereas the bilingual group was composed of 56 bilinguals who spoke English and one of eighteen non-English at home: Italian (9), Spanish (7), Arabic(6), Russian (5), Urdu (5), Mandarin (4), Cantonese (3), French (3), Hebrew (3), Persian (2),Tamil (2), Amharic (1), Hindi (1), Hungarian (1), Portuguese (1),

Punjabi (1), Romanian (1), or Serbian (1). Although bilingual advantage was found for these bilinguals on the three tests of executive functioning (Luria's tapping task measuring response inhibition, the Opposite Worlds task requiring children to assign incongruent labels to a sequence of animal pictures, and reverse categorization in which children needed to reclassify a set of objects into incongruent categories after an initial classification), these bilinguals were obviously from different L1 and cultural background.

More studies have examined bilingual advantage by testing participants who were immigrants with different L1s and cultural backgrounds. As in Bialystok and Viswanathan (2009), the bilinguals were educated in English and spoke another language at home: Cantonese, Croatian, French, Hebrew, Hindi, Kannada, Mandarin, Marati, Punjabi, Russian, Tagalog, Telugu, or Urdu (Bialystok & Viswanathan, 2009). Although positive evidence was found for bilingual advantage, the variety of these different languages and their respective cultural backgrounds remain a significant confounding factor. One typical study (Tao et al., 2011) examined Chinese-English bilinguals and English monolinguals and found a significant advantage for the bilinguals in conflict resolution, but the late Chinese-English bilinguals were only immigrants (30, Mandarin and Cantonese) in Australia, thus having different cultural and L1 background from the English monolinguals.

Among the studies that fail to capture bilingual advantage, for example in a study recently conducted by Paap and Greenberg (2013), it is found that there is no coherence for a bilingual advantage in executive processing. But in the study, the 122 bilinguals spoke 30 different languages (Spanish or Cantonese or Mandarin or Tagalog etc. as the first language and English as the second language), whereas the monolinguals were English-speaking native speakers. After testing the participants on tasks such as the Flanker, the Simon, and the Color-shape Switching, bilingual advantage was not observed at all. Similarly, the bilingual participants were immigrant bilinguals who had heterogeneous L1s and cultural backgrounds.

In all, whether bilingual advantage is found or not, bilinguals and their matched monolinguals are usually not homogenous in their L1s and cultural bearings. The distance between bilinguals' first language and second language will very likely modulate the interference between languages, thus leading to bilingual advantage to different degrees. In one such study (van Heuven et al., 2011), it turns out that for bilingual groups with different language scripts (e.g., Arabic, Chinese, and alphabetic in Uyghur-Chinese-English trilinguals), the magnitude of within-language Stroop interference is similar, whereas between-language Stroop interference is modulated by cross-language similarity. Moreover, cultural bearings may be another confounding factor. If participants are mixed with cultural differences, such differences will probably contribute to the variations of cognitive control performance; therefore, it is difficult to see clearly the nature of bilingual advantage. A recent study of cultural differences in human brain activity (Han & Ma, 2014) shows that social cognitive processes are characterized by stronger activity in the dorsal medial prefrontal cortex, lateral frontal cortex and temporoparietal junction in East Asians (Chinese, Japanese, Korea) but stronger activity in the anterior cingulate, ventral medial prefrontal cortex and bilateral insula in Westerners (Americans and Europeans). Moreover, East Asian cultures are associated with increased neural activity in the brain regions related to inference of others' mind and emotion regulation whereas Western cultures are associated with enhanced neural activity in the brain areas related to self-relevance encoding and emotional responses during social cognitive/affective processes. If culture modulates cognitive processes, it potentially confounds previous findings concerning bilingual advantage when recruited participants are from different cultural backgrounds.

Therefore, if we want to investigate bilingual advantage among a particular group of bilinguals, for example Chinese-English bilinguals, it is necessary for us to include monolinguals from the same cultural background of the bilinguals. As more and more Chinese are learning one or more foreign languages (particularly English) from primary education through higher education due to the open-up policy, investigating bilingual samples from the Chinese context is of great importance and may provide a more general picture painting the relationship between bilingualism and cognitive control.

Moreover, most previous studies adopted only one single behavioral task which usually tested just one aspect of cognitive control. As we have stated in earlier chapters, cognitive control can be decomposed into different aspects, such as inhibition, conflict monitoring, mental set shifting, working memory updating…, which are relevant but relatively independent to each other (Miyake et al., 2000). Therefore, testing only one aspect of cognitive control (such as only by Flanker or Simon task to test inhibition) can not tell us the full picture of bilingual advantage. As pointed out by Paap and Greenberg (2013), although previous studies adopt different tasks in different studies, the same set of matched bilinguals and monolinguals typically participate in only a single task, hence, providing only a single measure of certain aspect of cognitive control.

Therefore, in the current experiment (***Experiment One***), we examine whether there is a bilingual advantage among young adult Chinese-English bilinguals in the Chinese context, in which bilinguals and monolinguals share the same demographic, cultural, and L1 background (with their L2 – English as a foreign language). The homogeneity of the Chinese-English bilinguals and the Chinese monolinguals in native language, culture, and demographic features provides a purer situation to examine bilingual advantage. If bilingual advantage is genuine and general, it should also be found among the Chinese-English bilingual populations. Moreover, as stated earlier, a single task only measures mainly one single aspect of cognitive control, so multiple tasks are adopted in the current experiment for a more objective and all-round investigation of bilingual advantage. For these two purposes, two homogeneous groups of young adult Chinese participants (bilinguals and monolinguals) are required to complete three different tasks – the Flanker, the Number Stroop, and the WCST (Wisconsin Card Sorting Test) – that measure three different aspects of cognitive control, including conflict monitoring, conflict resolution/inhibition, and mental set shifting. As discussed in the previous review, these three aspects have been reported much relevant to bilingualism. Numerous studies have tapped these aspects that may be enhanced by bilingual experience (e.g., see Bialystok et al., 2009 for a review).

4.3 Method

4.3.1 Participants

There were altogether seventy-six participants in the experiment, with a mean age of 21.99 years (SD=2.740), 19 males and 57 females. All the participants took part in this experiment either for monetary compensation or for course credit. All of them reported normal or corrected-to-normal vision and had no speech or hearing disorders. They gave informed consent and their rights were protected in accordance with the ethical standards of the Academic Board from the bilinguals' university.

The bilinguals were native speakers of Chinese, composed of 43 English-major undergraduate/graduate students from a university in China. The 33 monolinguals, who had been working for around 5 years, graduated from junior, senior or vocational school where they learnt very limited English. More critically, their English proficiency was extremely low and they were not able to use any English in daily life/work at all. For the current research purpose we define them as monolinguals although a few reported extremely limited knowledge of English[1]. A questionnaire was administered for both groups with the purpose to collect the participants' demographic and educational background and language experience (Marian, Blumenfeld, & Kaushanskaya, 2007). L2 proficiency[2], composed of listening, speaking, reading, and writing, was self-rated on a 10-point Likert scale, which is a widely recognized measurement in bilingual research and is significantly correlated with objective measurements of language proficiency (Marian et al., 2007; Prior & Gollan, 2011). In

1 It's an acceptable practice that participants with an extremely limited knowledge of L2 are regarded as monolinguals, as in Prior and Macwhinney (2010) and in Paap and Greenberg (2013) etc. Furthermore, pure monolinguals are actually rare as nowadays individuals more or less have some knowledge of another language or dialect even though they are not able to use it.

2 We assumed that both the bilingual group and the monolingual group were homogenous in L1 since L1 was their native language and they were proficient enough to conduct successful and fluent communication. We believe that there was no significant difference in their L1 proficiency although there might be variations, such as the fact that bilinguals might have a disadvantage in L1 vocabulary size and fluency (Bialystok et al., 2009; Bialystok et al., 2010).

the scale, "1" indicates knowing nothing of the language and "10" indicates having a perfect master of the language. As objective test of L2 proficiency, both groups of participants took the test of English Verbal Fluency, in which participants were required to produce as many words as possible according to the presented category (jobs, sports, animals) in 60 seconds. Category fluency is reported to be strongly indicative of vocabulary size (Bialystok et al., 2009). For Intelligence measurement, all participants took the Ravens Advanced Progressive Matrices (Raven, Court, & Raven, 1977) (Chinese revised version). The task consists of 72 items, which are grouped in six types, and in each type there are 12 items. Each item is composed of a pattern with a missing part in the lower right. Participants were required to select the right one from a set of six or eight alternatives to complete the pattern within 40 minutes. Correct numbers of answers were calculated as original intelligence scores (not transformed into Chinese norm as we only needed to clarify that participants were homogeneous groups within the young adult age range). Table 1 lists the major characteristics[3] between the two groups.

Table 1. Participant characteristics in language history and background etc. between monolingual group and bilingual group.

	Monolingual n=33		*Bilingual n=43*		*(t-test) p value*
	Mean	*SD*	*Mean*	*SD*	
Age	21.5	3.6	22.4	1.8	.175
Education (years)	11.3	2.4	16.4	1.8	.000
Raven's Matrices*	65.2	5.5	64.7	4.1	.710
L2 Learning History	4.1	1.2	12.4	1.7	.000
L2 Proficiency*	7.1	2.9	24.8	2.9	.000
L2 Verbal Fluency	6.7	1.7	24.4	4.2	.000

Note: * Scores of Raven's Matrices were original intelligence scores and not transformed into Chinese norm as we only needed to clarify that participants were homogeneous groups within the young adult age range. The total score for L2 proficiency is 40.

3 We did not assess participants' social economic status (SES) because they were not so much relevant to our participants in the present study. Although Hook et al. (2013) suggested an association between SES and cognitive control, this association is mostly based on child bilinguals (but see Prior & Gollan, 2011). What's more, the participants in the present study came from similar family background. Thus we assumed that there was no systematic SES bias across the groups.

To summarize, there were two major characteristics between the bilingual group and the monolingual group. Firstly, the monolingual group had extremely limited proficiency of English (which was a foreign language to them) and basically had no chance of being exposed to English use or speaking in their life. However, the bilinguals were undergraduates or graduates in English major. They had significantly longer time of English learning and higher English proficiency (self-rated and objective test) and used English quite more often in their study and daily life. Secondly, although the monolinguals and the bilinguals differed in the time of education they had received ($p<.001$), the two groups were matched on IQ and age, both of whom were young adults with the mean age from 21.5 to 22.4.

4.3.2 Materials and Procedure

Three computerized tasks were administered to measure participants' cognitive control. The tasks, which included the Flanker task, the Number Stroop task, and the Wisconsin Card Sorting Test (WCST), were designed to test cognitive control in three different aspects: conflict monitoring, inhibitory control/inhibition, and mental set shifting. The first dependent variable we investigated is the response times in each condition of the Flanker task and the Number Stroop task. The response times of each condition in these two tasks indicate participants' ability of conflict monitoring. A faster response time in each condition reflects a stronger ability of conflict monitoring (Costa et al., 2009; Paap & Greenberg, 2013). The second dependent variable we tested is the conflict effect, which is the difference in response times between congruent trials and incongruent trials in these two tasks. A smaller difference in response times reflects a stronger ability of conflict resolution, thus a stronger ability of inhibitory control/inhibition (Bialystok et al., 2009; Costa et al., 2009; Paap & Greenberg, 2013). The third dependent variable we measured is the performance of the WCST, reflected by global RTs, completed categories, overall errors, and types of errors as the characteristics of this task. A better performance indicates a stronger ability of mental set shifting (Miyake et al., 2000; Yudes et al., 2011).

In this experiment, which lasted for approximately 1.5 hours, participants firstly completed a set of composite questionnaires tapping on their language and demographic background, and secondly completed the three computerized cognitive control tasks.

Cognitive Control Tasks

Flanker Task

The Flanker task (Eriksen & Eriksen, 1974) is used to assess one's ability to suppress responses that are inappropriate in a particular context (Festman & Munte, 2012; Luk et al., 2010). In this test, participants are instructed to respond to the direction of a red target chevron that is surrounded by various other symbols. Presented in Figure 16 are samples of different Flanker trials in three conditions: neutral, congruent and incongruent conditions. In neutral trials, the flanking stimuli are black diamonds presenting no relevant information to the target chevron. In congruent trials, the target chevron is flanked by four black chevrons pointing in the same direction as the target. In incongruent trials, the four flanking chevrons point in the direction opposite to that indicated by the target, creating conflict and interference.

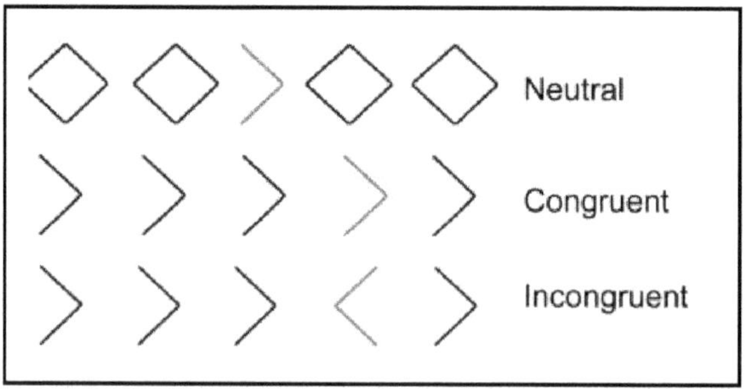

Figure 16. Sample stimuli in the three conditions of the Flanker task.

The computerized task, programmed in E-prime (version 2.0), consists of a practice block with 9 trials (with feedback) and the experimental block, which includes 108 trials. The experimental block will not start until each participant reaches a correction rate above 80% in the practice block. Each trial starts with a fixation of "+" for 250ms. Then an experimental stimulus is randomly presented for 2000 ms or until designated keys are pressed.

Number Stroop Task

The Stroop Interference Test (Stroop, 1935), similar to the Flanker task, is used to measure participants' ability to inhibit an over-learned (i.e., dominant) response in favor of an unusual one (Spreen & Strauss, 1998). The number-Stroop paradigm (Bush et al., 1998; Girelli, Sandrini, Cappa, & Butterworth, 2001; Tzelgov, Meyer, & Henik, 1992), requires participants to decide whether the number of stimuli presented is odd or even. In neutral trials, the stimuli are shapes of the pound sign "#". For example, if it is "###", the number of the stimulus is 3, so it is odd. In both congruent and incongruent trials, the stimuli are digits. In congruent trials, the number of the digits coincides with the digit itself, such as in the case of "333". In incongruent trials, the number of the digits causes interference when odd or even shall be decided, such as in the case of "3333" (Figure 17).

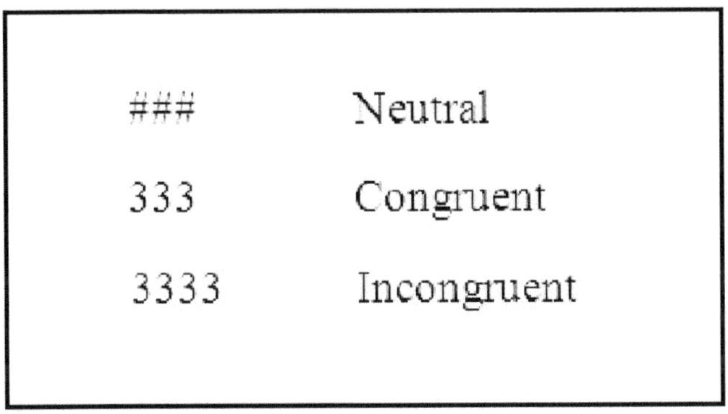

Figure 17. Example of the three conditions in the Number Stroop Task.

As in the Flanker task, the computerized Number Stroop test consists of two blocks: the practice block and the experimental block. There are 9 trials in the practice block, in which feedback of accuracy and response times are presented, and there are 120 formal trials randomly presented in the experimental block, in which no feedback is given. Each stimulus is presented for a maximum time of 2000 ms or until participants respond by pressing designated keys. Participants are required to respond as quickly as possible without sacrificing accuracy.

Wisconsin Card Sorting Test (WCST)

The WCST is used to detect participant's ability to infer the implied rule in card sorting and to switch their mental sets. The present experiment follows procedures from previous studies (Festman & Munte, 2012; Yudes et al., 2011). The test is composed of 128 response-cards and 4 stimulus-cards depicting different dimensions of geometric figures. The first dimension is the number of items: one, two, three, or four; the second dimension color: red, green, yellow, or blue; the third shape: triangle, star, cross, or circle. Each response card has a combination of three dimensions, like the example card of **Four Green Crosses** in Figure 18. The 4 stimulus cards respectively depict one red triangle, two green stars, three yellow crosses, and four blue circles. Participants are required to sort each response card according to only one dimension of the 4 stimulus cards (by pressing designated key). The participants receive information on whether their responses are correct or not, but they are not informed about the underlying rule, which will change after a few trials (from 5 to 9). For example in Figure 18, if the underlying rule is number, then the correct response is pressing the button representing the last stimulus card – four blue circles. If the underlying rule is shape, then the correct response is pressing the third stimulus card – three yellow crosses.

In the computerized version, participants are required to sort the card by pressing the designated button that indicates an implied rule. There are 12 practice trials in the practice block and 128 formal trials in the experimental block. Participants will not go into the experimental block until they fully understand what to do. There is a fixation of 1000 ms before a stimulus appears. The stimulus lasts for no more than 3000 ms, in which participants have to respond by pressing designated keys (one key for each dimension). Participants receive feedback (1000ms) of "correct" or "incorrect" for their response. The experiment proceeds in this way until all the 128 cards are completed.

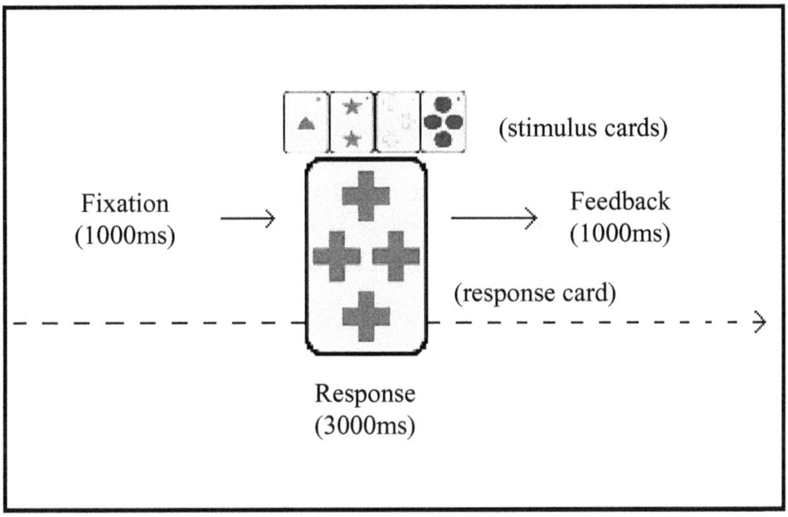

Figure 18. Example of stimulus presentation of the WCST.

4.4 Result

4.4.1 Data Trimming

Firstly, in the tasks of Flanker and Number Stroop, data of erroneous and extreme responses were firstly excluded. Secondly, in all the tasks, trials that fell above 3 standard deviations (SDs) of the overall mean response times (RTs) for each subject in each condition were then eliminated, accounting for 2.37% of the total correct responses. Thirdly, in the WCST task, besides global RTs, completed categories, overall errors and types of errors were analyzed respectively to investigate group differences.

4.4.2 Flanker Task

Table 2 presents the data for the Flanker task between the two groups. One participant from the monolingual group was excluded because of false operations in the task. Two indices were used to compare between-group performances. The first one is Flanker conflict, the difference in mean response times between trials that require conflict resolution (incongruent) compared with those that do not (congruent). Smaller Flanker conflict implies superior ability in conflict resolution, thus stronger ability of inhibition (Bialystok et al., 2004; Bialystok, Craik, & Luk, 2008; Costa et al., 2009; Paap & Greenberg, 2013). The second one is the mean RTs in each condition, which reflects global goal-oriented maintenance and conflict monitoring. Faster RTs in the task indicates superior performance in conflict monitoring. Bilingual advantage in overall RTs may reveal bilinguals' better ability to handle tasks that involve mixing trials of different types, i.e. the efficiency of monitoring system (Costa et al., 2009; Costa et al., 2008; Martin-Rhee & Bialystok, 2008).

Table 2. Means and standard deviations of response times in Flanker conditions and Flanker conflict between monolingual group and bilingual group.

	Monolingual n=32		*Bilingual n=43*		*p value*
	Mean	*SD*	*Mean*	*SD*	*(t-test)*
Flanker Neutral	549.3	90.8	536.0	91.3	.535
Flanker Incongruent	589.7	88.3	578.3	87.1	.581
Flanker Congruent	530.3	106.4	516.4	80.6	.522
Flanker Conflict*	59.4	39.7	61.9	49.5	.806

Note: *Flanker conflict means the different response times between incongruent condition and congruent condition.

We conducted a repeated measures analysis of variance (ANOVA) with Group (the monolingual group, the bilingual group) as between-subject variable and Condition (neutral, incongruent, congruent) as within-subject variable. This analysis revealed a significant main effect of Condition, F (2, 146) =79.651, p<.001, η^2=.522, but there was no Condition and Group interaction (F<1). Planned comparisons showed that participants responded more quickly on the neutral condition (541.68) than on the incongruent condition (583.16), F (1, 73) =86.703, p<.001. Participants responded more quickly on the congruent condition (522.31) than on the neutral condition (541.68), F (1, 73) =15.353, p<.001, and than on the incongruent condition (583.16), F (1, 73) =130.037, p<.001, reflecting significant Flanker effect (the RT difference between congruent and incongruent trials). However, the main effect of Group was not significant, F (1, 73) =.398, p=.530, η^2=.005. There were no differences between the monolingual group and the bilingual group in the three conditions of the Flanker task. Furthermore, independent sample t-test of the Flanker conflict effect revealed that there was no group difference between the monolinguals and the bilinguals (p=.806).

This analysis of the group performance in the Flanker task suggests that the young adult Chinese-English bilingual group does not exhibit bilingual advantage compared with the monolingual group, either in the aspect of conflict monitoring or in the aspect of inhibition.

4.4.3 Number Stroop Task

The Number Stroop Task, which cognitively requires higher demands than the Flanker task, was also used to measure the two aspects of cognitive control: conflict monitoring and conflict effect. Table 3 lists the data of this task performance between the two groups. Four participants from the two groups were excluded because of false operations. We expected that the bilingual group might be better in performing this task compared with the monolingual group.

Like what we did in analyzing the Flanker task performance, the same indices (global RTs and Stroop conflict) were compared in order to examine the performance differences between the two groups. Similarly, a repeated measures analysis of variance (ANOVA) was conducted with Group (the monolingual group, the bilingual group) as between-subject variable and Condition (neutral, incongruent, congruent) as within-subject variable. This analysis revealed a significant main effect of Condition, F (2, 140) =14.237, p<.001, η^2=.169, but there was no Condition and Group interaction, F (2, 140) =1.009, p=.367, η^2=.014. Planned comparisons showed that participants did not respond more quickly on the neutral condition (729.80) than on the incongruent condition (723.99), $F<1$, but participants responded more quickly on the congruent condition (693.49) than on the neutral condition (729.80), $F(1,70)=31.507, p<.001$, and than on the incongruent condition (723.99), $F(1, 70)=17.353$, $p<.001$, reflecting significant Stroop conflict effect (the RT difference between congruent and incongruent trials).

Table 3. Means and standard deviations of reaction times in the Number Stroop conditions, means and standard deviations of Stroop conflict between monolingual group and bilingual group.

	Monolingual *n=31*		*Bilingual* *n=41*		*p value*
	Mean	*SD*	*Mean*	*SD*	*(t-test)*
Number Stroop Neutral	721.8	119.3	735.9	107.9	.601
Number Stroop Incongruent	712.5	95.2	732.7	98.3	.386
Number Stroop Congruent	693.2	100.0	693.7	95.9	.982
Number Stroop Conflict*	19.3	50.7	39.0	63.2	.167

Note: *Number Stroop conflict means the different response times between incongruent condition and congruent condition.

However, the main effect of Group was not significant, $F<1$. There were no differences between the monolingual group and the bilingual group in the three conditions of the Number Stroop task. Moreover, independent sample *t*-test of the Number Stroop conflict effect revealed that there was no group difference between the monolinguals and the bilinguals ($p=.167$).

The results of the Number Stroop task are similar to those of the Flanker task performed by the bilingual group and the monolingual group. On the aspects of conflict monitoring and inhibitory control (inhibition), compared with the counterpart Chinese monolinguals, no positive evidence is found for a bilingual advantage among the young adult Chinese-English bilinguals.

4.4.4 WCST

Different from the Flanker task and the Number Stroop task, the WCST task was used to test participants' ability of mental set shifting in cognitive control. Better performance of the WCST task indicates superior ability in mental set shifting. In executing the task, participants had to keep switching from one rule to another and at the same time inhibit the prepotent response of using previous rule, that is to say, the ability to disengage an irrelevant task set and subsequently engage a relevant task set (Miyake et al., 2000). To capture the performance differences in mental flexibility between groups, the performance indicators we measured included global performance (global RTs, number of completed categories and number of errors) and local performance (different types of errors: perseverative errors, previous category errors) (Barceló & Knight, 2002; Yudes et al., 2011). The bilingual group might perform better than the monolingual group since the bilinguals had a constant need to switch from one language to the other, while the monolinguals had not. The means and standard deviations of the global RTs, the number of completed categories, overall errors, perseverative errors, and previous category errors between groups are presented in Table 4. One participant from the monolingual group was excluded because of false operations.

To compare the between-group differences in the WCST task performance, an independent sample *t*-test was conducted. We analyzed two broad categories of the WCST performance: global performance (global RTs, completed categories, overall errors) and local performance (types of errors: perseverative errors, previous category errors).

The result of global RTs showed that there was no difference in terms of response times in the WCST performance between the monolingual group and the bilingual group. The second indicator of global performance was the number of completed categories. In this version of WCST, there were 19 categories altogether, with "0" indicating that the participant was not able to complete at least five consecutive correct responses to trials of any category. "19" indicates that the participant completed trials of all the categories. The result of independent sample t-test on the number of completed categories showed that there was significant difference between the monolingual group and the bilingual group (p<.001), with the bilingual group (9.2 categories) completing a significantly higher number of categories than the monolingual group (5.7 categories).

Table 4. Means and standard deviations of global RTs, completed categories, overall errors, perseverative errors, and previous category errors between monolingual group and bilingual group.

	Monolingual n=32		*Bilingual n=43*		*p value*
	Mean	*SD*	*Mean*	*SD*	*(t-test)*
Global RTs	1383.7	549.8	1555.5	526.3	.178
Completed categories	5.7	2.8	9.2	3.4	.000
Overall errors	73.2	13.4	57.7	14.1	.000
Perseverative errors	54.4	15.4	37.3	15.3	.000
Previous category errors	41.6	17.7	19.9	13.1	.000

In terms of overall errors, the independent sample *t*-test showed that the monolingual group (73.2) committed significantly more errors than the bilingual group (57.7) (p<.001). The analysis of global performance in the WCST showed that the bilingual group performed significantly better than the monolingual group.

As for the types of errors, previous literature discriminates perseverative errors and non-perseverative errors (Heaton et al., 1993). When participants fail to change the mental rule after receiving negative feedback and continued sorting the cards according to previous category dimension(s), they commit perseverative errors (Yudes et al., 2011). In making perseverative errors, participants commit either perseverations to the immediately preceding category (previous category errors) or perseverations to a different category. Previous category perseverations reflect lack of flexibility to change the mental set to a new rule, while different category perseverations reflect the understanding that the previous rule is no longer correct but there is an unsuccessful attempt to infer a new rule (Hartman, Bolton, & Fehnel, 2001; Hartman, Steketee, Silva, Lanning, & Andersson, 2003; Yudes et al., 2011).

An independent sample t-test was conducted to compare the group differences in these types of errors. The results showed that the bilingual group (37.3) committed significantly fewer errors than the monolingual group (54.4) ($p<.001$) on perseverative errors. On previous category errors, independent sample t-test showed that there was significant difference ($p<.001$) between the monolingual group (41.6) and the bilingual group (19.9).

As shown in Table 1, the bilingual group and the monolingual group differed in the years of received education. In order to exclude the differences of this factor, we included education as a covariate to do ANCOVA analysis. The results showed that education years did not contribute significantly to the group differences in all the indices of the WCST task (global RT, $p=.663$; completed category, $p=.301$; overall errors, $p=.293$; perseverative errors, $p=.279$; previous category errors, $p=.326$), while group type contributed significantly to differences in the WCST performance (global RT, $p=.603$; completed category, $p=.032$; overall errors, $p=.030$; perseverative errors, $p=.033$; previous category errors, $p=.003$).

The performances in the WCST task support the theory that bilinguals have advantage over monolinguals in cognitive control. In the current experiment, the bilingual group and the monolingual group executed the task equally quickly, but the bilingual group completed more categories, committed fewer overall errors, fewer perseverative errors and fewer previous category errors than the monolingual group. These results robustly provide novel support for bilingual advantage among the young adult unbalanced Chinese-English bilinguals in the Chinese context.

4.5 Discussion

The goal of the current experiment is to test the hypothesis that bilingual experience leads to advantage in cognitive control among bilinguals, compared with their counterpart monolinguals. In the current experiment, we tested a group of young adult Chinese monolinguals and a group of young adult Chinese-English bilinguals, both of whom were homogeneous in L1, demographic and cultural background. We compared their cognitive control abilities in three aspects that had been mostly examined in previous literature: conflict monitoring, inhibition, and mental set shifting, through administering multiple tasks: the Flanker task, the Number Stroop task, and the WCST task.

The results are very clear. The young adult Chinese-English bilinguals show similar conflict monitoring and inhibition abilities to those of their Chinese monolingual peers (as tested in the Flanker and the Number Stroop). However, the young adult Chinese-English bilinguals show superior ability of mental set shifting compared with their Chinese counterpart monolinguals (as tested in the WCST). These results provide further evidence of bilingual advantage in cognitive control among the young adult Chinese-English bilinguals, but only in the aspect of mental set shifting.

There is a difference in cognitive demand between the Flanker task and the Number Stroop task (as reflected in the response times). As stated in the task design, the Number Stroop task requires the participants to monitor the context composed of two different dimensions (numbers and the oddness of numbers) and to inhibit the interference information/response from the other dimension, but in the Flanker task only one dimension (spatial direction) is required. However, in both the Flanker task and the Number Stroop task, no differences between the monolingual group and the bilingual group are found, either on the indicator of global RTs in the three conditions of each task or on the indicator of conflict effect in each task. The bilingual group does not outperform the monolingual group in the Flanker task and the Number Stroop task in the global RTs, indicating that the bilingual group is not superior to the monolingual group in terms of conflict monitoring, the ability to manage attention to a complex set of rapidly changing task demands (Bialystok et al., 2004), or the ability to handle tasks that involve mixing trials of different types (Costa et al., 2009). The bilingual group did not outperform the monolingual group either, in terms of conflict effect in each task, indicating that the bilingual group is not better than the monolingual group in the ability of conflict resolution, which reflects the ability to inhibit the misleading information or prepotent response (Paap & Greenberg, 2013). These results are contradictory to our prediction and previous findings that bilinguals have advantage over monolinguals in cognitive control tasks, particularly among the child and older adult bilinguals (Bialystok, 2010; Bialystok et al., 2004; Bialystok et al., 2005; Tao et al., 2011).

However, the results of the Flanker task and the Number Stroop task are actually consistent with some previous findings that young adult bilinguals show a modest or null effect of bilingual advantage compared with their counterparts (Bialystok et al., 2008; Kousaie & Phillips, 2012a; Paap & Greenberg, 2013). This can be explained by a few main reasons.

Firstly, the null effect of bilingual advantage among young adult bilinguals has often been attributed to the fact that young adult bilinguals are at the peak of cognitive control development, so they probably are able to perform the tasks (such as the Flanker and the Number Stroop) at the highest efficiency. Thus bilingualism provides no further boost (Bialystok et al., 2009; Bialystok et al., 2012). As mentioned earlier, there are more positive evidence of bilingual advantage among child bilinguals and older adult bilinguals (e.g., Bialystok et al., 2004; Bialystok et al., 2005; Bialystok et al., 2007), but among young adult bilinguals several studies have produced null effect (e.g., Paap & Greenberg, 2013). However, this explanation is not adequate because a few studies have also observed evidence of bilingual advantage in inhibition among young adult bilinguals (Prior & Gollan, 2011; Prior & Macwhinney, 2010; Tao et al., 2011).

Secondly, task demand may be another factor that modulates the effect. Bilingual advantage may not be observable if measuring task consumes low cognitive resources. In Costa et al. (2009), different versions of ANT task were designed and the result found that bilingual advantage was observable only in the difficult version where 50–50 percent of congruent trial and incongruent trials were mixed; whereas in the current experiment the trials were presented randomly. It is still possible that in more difficult task testing conflict control or monitoring, bilingual advantage will emerge. However, in the Number Stroop task, which is cognitively more demanding than the flanker task, there was no effect either.

Thirdly, the result that bilinguals are not superior to monolinguals in the aspects of conflict monitoring and inhibition might be attributed to the possibility that bilinguals did not engage much in monitoring or inhibition related language use experience. Suppose, for example, bilinguals use language in a context where inhibition is highly and intensively required, the effect might be statistically significant.

However, the null effect of bilingual advantage in these two tasks (Flanker and Number Stroop) does not rule out the possibility that the young adult Chinese-English bilingual group may outperform the Chinese monolingual group on other aspect(s) of cognitive control (e.g., mental set shifting), since cognitive control is composed of different and independent subcomponents as we have stated in previous sections.

The results of the WCST show that bilinguals are significantly better than monolinguals in mental set shifting. This is within our expectation in that bilinguals have intensive need to switch between two languages (which underlies the mechanism of mental set shifting) whereas the monolinguals do not have such need at all. A long term practice of switching between languages may, very probably, lead to the enhancement of mental set shifting in cognitive control. This result is also consistent or partly consistent with some previous findings that bilinguals outperform monolinguals in color-shape task switch or dimensional card sorting (e.g., Bialystok & Martin, 2004; Prior & Macwhinney, 2010; Prior & Gollan, 2011). However, in Paap and Greenberg (2013)'s study, no effect was found in the color-shape task switch, which also tested mental set shifting, probably because the task they adopted (color-shape task switch) was not demanding enough for their participants (Paap & Greenberg, 2013). The Color-shape task switch requires two dimensions, while the current task WCST requires three dimensions (color, shape, and number). Moreover, their participants were heterogeneous from different demographic and L1 backgrounds, whereas our participants were homogenous in demographic and linguistic background under the Chinese context.

Overall, the current experiment ***(Experiment One)*** results show no group differences in conflict monitoring or inhibition, but show group differences in mental set shifting. These results indicate that bilingual advantage is present, but only in a certain specific aspect (mental set shifting) of cognitive control, probably as a combined result of factors including age, task demand, and specific bilingual language use experience.

However, in literature, the origins and nature of bilingual advantage in cognitive control have remained largely unexplained. Bilingual advantage observed in child bilinguals, older adult bilinguals, and a few samples of young adult bilinguals have been considered the consequence of bilingual experience through which bilinguals monitor the language use context, inhibit the non-target language, and switch between two languages. If these origins are genuine, after matching the linguistic and demographic background between monolinguals and bilinguals, identify and classify specific bilingual experiences that may cause the enhancement of specific aspect of cognitive control should be crucial to reveal the nature of bilingual advantage in future research. That is, focus on how specific aspects of bilingual experience link to specific enhancement of cognitive control (Paap, 2014).

4.6 Conclusion

In conclusion, the current experiment results provide data showing that young adult Chinese-English bilinguals are similar to Chinese monolinguals in conflict monitoring and inhibiting, but they are more able to flexibly change from one mental set to another, i.e., a stronger ability of mental set shifting. These data provide further evidence clearly demonstrating that bilinguals have cognitive control advantage over monolinguals, which indicate that bilingual advantage is genuine and general. However, this advantage may be present only in some specific aspects. The reason for such specificity may come from a certain specific needs/experience involved in bilingual language processing, which will be further examined in the following chapters.

Chapter 5: Experiment Two – L2 Proficiency and Cognitive Control

5.1 Introduction

Although previous studies present us with a mixed picture of bilingual advantage among young adult bilinguals, **Experiment One** has indeed provided evidence of bilingual advantage that young-adult unbalanced Chinese-English bilinguals have advantage in cognitive control compared with their Chinese counterpart monolinguals. However, their bilingual advantage is limited only in the aspect of mental set shifting but not in conflict monitoring or inhibiting. **Experiment One** does give further support for bilingual advantage, but it still does not tell us which specific aspects of bilingual experiences may have caused this bilingual advantage? As discussed in *Chapter Three*, different types of bilingual experiences, such as different L2 proficiency and language use, may lead to variations of bilingual advantage in cognitive control. The current experiment (**Experiment Two**) is to answer *Research Question 2*: *Does language (L2) proficiency contribute to cognitive control differences among young-adult bilinguals?*

5.2 Specific Background

As already mentioned in *Chapter Three*, most previous studies do not take into account that there are different types of bilinguals, differing in terms of such factors as their language proficiency (particularly L2) or in how they use the second language or how often they switch between the two languages etc. Moreover, most previous studies on bilingual advantage focus on cognitive control differences only between bilingual groups and monolingual groups (Bialystok et al., 2008; Prior & Macwhinney, 2010). There are at least two limitations for previous investigations.

First, the bilingual groups examined are heterogeneous in that bilinguals either speak a wide variety of language pairs or are single groups of highly balanced bilinguals (Colzato et al., 2008; Costa et al., 2008) or use languages in varied contexts (Green, 2011). The heterogeneity of bilingual groups, very likely, may result in variations of cognitive control ability.

Second, few designs allow for a direct comparison between different bilingual populations or an investigation of the degree to which one must be bilingual before exhibiting any advantage[4]. Therefore, it is difficult to identify precisely what about bilingualism is critical for the observed effect (Prior & Gollan, 2011).

As bilinguals vary greatly in their bilingual language experiences, it is reasonable to assume that these differences in bilingual experience will cause variations of bilingual advantage in cognitive control. We adhere to the view that the comparisons between bilinguals with different characteristics such as language proficiency can provide us with a significant perspective to look into which aspect of bilingualism contributes to bilingual advantage in cognitive control. By comparing different bilingual groups with different characteristics, we are able to see how specific features/aspects of bilingualism are related to cognitive control. The current experiment (**Experiment Two**) focuses on how one of the main features of bilingualism – L2 proficiency – is related to cognitive control.

A few recent studies suggest that language proficiency (particularly L2) may be an independent factor that affects cognitive control in bilinguals (Abutalebi et al., 2013; Iluz-Cohen & Armon-Lotem, 2013; Marian, Blumenfeld, Mizrahi, Kania, & Cordes, 2013; Pivneva, Palmer, & Titone, 2012). According to Tse and Altarriba (2012), bilinguals' first and second language proficiency modulates their performance in conflict resolution and goal maintenance while performing the Stroop

4 Only few recent studies have directly compared different bilingual groups in the study of bilingualism (Barac & Bialystok, 2012; Singh & Mishra, 2012; Tse & Altarriba, 2012), and the current research is a further contribution.

task (Tse & Altarriba, 2012). One more recent study shows that young bilinguals (19.5–22.1 years) with higher L2 proficiency react faster than lower L2 proficiency bilinguals in target detection tasks (Mishra, Hilchey, Singh, & Klein, 2012). Another recent study, which uses eye movement techniques to explore this issue, shows that bilinguals with higher L2 proficiency have a better oculomotor control compared with their lower L2 proficiency counterparts (Singh & Mishra, 2013). Moreover, via the attention network task, Videsott et al. (2012) suggest that linguistic competence (proficiency), rather than competence in other skill domains, has a decisive role in the alerting component of executive control (Videsott, Della Rosa, Wiater, Franceschini, & Abutalebi, 2012). Therefore, these studies positively indicate that there is a strong relationship between language proficiency (particularly L2 proficiency) and cognitive control.

However, from the above-mentioned literature regarding language proficiency and cognitive control, we recognize that the tasks (such as Stroop, target detection task, and ANT) adopted in the previous studies mainly measured the aspect of inhibition in cognitive control. As discussed earlier, however, cognitive control can be decomposed into several related but relatively independent aspects such as inhibition, mental set shifting, monitoring and updating etc. (Miyake & Friedman, 2012; Miyake et al., 2000). Thus a strong positive relationship between language proficiency and inhibition in cognitive control does not necessarily indicate a strong positive relationship between language proficiency and other aspects of cognitive control. Therefore, there are two purposes for the current experiment (**Experiment Two**): first, to verify whether second language (L2) proficiency differences between bilinguals will bring about different performances in cognitive control tasks measuring inhibition; second, to investigate whether second language (L2) proficiency may affect cognitive control in two other aspects – conflict monitoring and mental set shifting.

We investigate whether bilinguals with differing L2 proficiency levels will have significant differences in cognitive control by requiring them to perform the same tasks adopted by Experiment One: the Flanker task, the Number Stroop task, and the WCST task, which measured three aspects of cognitive control: conflict monitoring, inhibition, and mental set shifting. These tasks allow us to see more specifically the association between language proficiency and different aspect(s) of cognitive control by examining different bilingual groups differing in L2 proficiency. Specifically, for our investigation, we include two homogeneous groups of young-adult unbalanced Chinese-English bilinguals, who differ in L2 proficiency, for comparisons. We hypothesize that L2 proficiency will contribute significantly to the differences of bilingual advantage in cognitive control. The higher L2 proficiency bilinguals may perform better than the lower L2 proficiency bilinguals in some of the cognitive control tasks, or all the tasks.

5.3 Method

5.3.1 Participants

One hundred and five young-adult Chinese-English bilinguals (9 males/96 females, right-handed) with a mean age of 21.21 years (SD=1.645) participated in this experiment either for monetary compensation or for course credit. All of them were students from a university in mainland China. They all reported normal or corrected-to-normal vision and had no speech or hearing disorders. All participants gave informed consent and their rights were protected according to the ethics of the university Academic Board. The participants came from English major students of the university, and they were at the undergraduate level or at the graduate level of higher education.

To incorporate group differences, we required all the participants to report their background such as demographic characteristics, language proficiency and English (L2) learning history. The participants were divided into two groups according to their English learning background and L2 proficiency. L2 proficiency was firstly rated subjectively by a self-rating questionnaire (same as the one adopted in Experiment 1) (Marian et al., 2007). In the questionnaire, English (L2) proficiency was rated using a 10-point Likert Scale, with "1" indicating knowing nothing of the language and "10" indicating having a perfect master of the language. Four parts of L2 proficiency were rated: Speaking, Listening, Reading, and Writing. Secondly, as objective test of L2 proficiency[5], both groups of participants took the test of English Verbal Fluency (same as the one in Experiment 1), in which participants were required to produce as many words as possible according to the presented category (jobs, sports, animals) in 60 seconds. Category fluency is reported to be strongly indicative of vocabulary size (Bialystok et al., 2009). For objective test of Intelligence, all participants took Ravens Advanced Progressive Matrices (same as the one in Experiment 1) (Raven et al., 1977), which consists of 72 items grouped in six types. In each type there are 12 items. Each item is composed of a pattern with a missing part in the lower right. Participants were required to select the right one from a set of six or eight alternatives to complete the pattern within 40 minutes. Correct answers were counted as intelligence scores. The characteristics[6] of these two groups are presented in Table 5.

Table 5. Participant characteristics between bilinguals differing in L2 proficiency.

	Higher L2 group *n=43*		*Lower L2 group* *n=62*		*p value*
	M	*SD*	*M*	*SD*	*(t-test)*
Age	22.4	1.8	20.4	0.9	.000
Raven's Matrices	64.7	4.1	65.2	3.6	.537
English (L2) learning history	12.4	1.7	10.4	0.9	.000
English (L2) proficiency (1–10)	23.2	4.5	21.0	4.0	.014
L2 Verbal Fluency (category)	24.4	4.2	21.4	4.8	.001
English (L2) exposure (%)	43.3	17.7	44.7	21.6	.730

Note. For the percentage (%), Chinese and English equal 100 percent.

5 Only English proficiency was assessed. This is based on our presumption that our participants, who had passed college entrance examination and were regular college students majoring in English, must have maintained homogeneously a high proficiency of their native language – Mandarin Chinese. We believe that there was no systematic difference in their L1 proficiency (although there might be variations) due to the homogeneity of their educational background.

6 The participants in the current study came from similar family and educational background. Thus we assumed that there was no systematic SES bias between the groups.

As we can see from Table 5, the two groups differed significantly in age. However, it was not much relevant in our experiment because both groups were young adult bilinguals between 20.4–22.4 years old and both groups were in the peak of cognitive control development. The two groups differed significantly in English learning history (*ps*<.001). This is understandable that the higher L2 proficiency bilinguals[7] had been learning English for a longer time than the lower L2 proficiency bilinguals at school since both groups started learning English at around age 10. More importantly, between these two bilingual groups, the results of self-rated English proficiency and verbal fluency test consistently showed that the higher L2 proficiency group significantly differed from the lower L2 proficiency group in L2 proficiency (p=.014, p=.001 for self rating and verbal fluency respectively). Furthermore, the two demographically homogeneous groups were comparable in IQ and similar in English background such as English exposure (p>.05). Therefore, if there were some differences between the two groups in cognitive control, we would attribute them to L2 proficiency.

5.3.2 Materials and Procedure

All participants completed a battery of linguistic and cognitive measures in a quiet behavior lab room. Computerized tasks were programmed by software E-prime 2.0 on a desktop computer with 17-inch color monitor. Reaction times were recorded by pressing designated keys on computer keyboard. Participants were able to adjust their seat approximately 60cm from the monitor. In order to have measurement coherence, we adopted the same three cognitive tasks used in Experiment One. The tasks were designed to test three components of cognitive control: conflict monitoring, inhibition, and mental set shifting. The global RTs in different trial conditions from the Flanker task and the Number Stroop task reflect the ability of conflict monitoring (Costa et al., 2009), the conflict effect (RTs difference between the incongruent trials and congruent trials) in both the Flanker task and the Number Stroop task reflect the ability of inhibitory control/inhibition (Paap &

---

7 This group of bilinguals was the same bilingual group in Experiment One.

Greenberg, 2013), and the WCST performance overall reflect the ability of mental set shifting (Yudes et al., 2011).

Cognitive Control Tasks
The three behavioral tasks were identical to those in Experiment One.

5.4 Result

5.4.1 Data Trimming

Correct response times were analyzed by SPSS 15.0. Outliers and data deviating from 3SDs from the mean for each participant in each condition were trimmed separately for each task. In all for the Flanker task and the Number Stroop task, the data above and below 3SDs accounted for 2.33% of the total data. In the WCST task, we calculated the mean RTs for each of the subjects, and excluded extremes and trials that fell 3 SDs above or below the mean RTs (1.86%). We then counted the characteristic indexes of the WSCT task for each participant, including completed categories, overall errors and types of errors.

5.4.2 Flanker Task

To determine whether bilinguals of higher L2 proficiency would complete the Flanker task more efficiently than bilinguals of lower L2 proficiency, we conducted repeated measures analysis of variance with language group (higher L2 group, lower L2 group) as between subject variable and condition (congruent, neutral, and incongruent) as within subject variables. Table 6 lists the data of mean RTs and SDs of each group in the Flanker task. In the Flanker task, one participant was excluded because of false operations.

Table 6. Mean reaction times, Flanker conflict, and standard deviations in the Flanker task between groups differing in L2.

	Higher L2 group n=43		*Lower L2 group n=61*		*p value*
	M	*SD*	*M*	*SD*	*(t-test)*
Flanker neutral	536.0	91.3	527.9	94.6	.662
Flanker incongruent	578.3	87.1	566.9	101.7	.552
Flanker congruent	516.3	80.6	511.7	109.3	.815
Flanker conflict*	62.0	49.5	55.2	35.3	.415

Note. *Flanker conflict refers to the RT difference between incongruent and congruent conditions.

In the analysis of the Flanker task performance, the main effect of condition was significant, F (2,204) =107.688; p<.001; η^2=.514. Planned comparisons showed that participants responded more quickly in the congruent condition (513.68 ms) than in the neutral (531.24 ms) and incongruent conditions (571.63 ms) (ps<.001), and participants responded more quickly in the neutral condition (531.24 ms) than in the incongruent condition (571.63 ms) (p<.001), reflecting a significant Flanker conflict effect (RT difference between congruent and incongruent condition). However, the analysis revealed no main effect of participant group F (1,102) =.189, p=.664, and the interaction between participant group and Flanker condition was not significant F (2,204) =.346, p=.708, reflecting that there was no group difference in the speed and efficiency in performing the three conditions of the Flanker task. Moreover, an independent sample t-test analysis showed that there was no group difference in terms of the Flanker conflict (RTs difference between congruent and incongruent condition) between groups (p=.415), reflecting that the two groups did not differ in conflict resolution when congruent and incongruent trials were mixed.

To conclude, as can be seen in Table 5, the two groups had similar English learning background such as L2 exposure; however, the two groups differed significantly in L2 proficiency, as indicated by self-rated questionnaire and verbal fluency test (p=.014, p=.001 respectively). So if there were any differences in the Flanker task performance, we would attribute them to the difference of L2 proficiency. However, there were no group differences either in speed or in conflict effect in performing the Flanker task.

In order to further clarify the role of L2 proficiency in the Flanker task performance, however, we conducted multiple regression analysis by entering L2 proficiency, age, L2 history, and L2 exposure as independent variables. The results showed that the multiple regression models (*F*s<1) were nonsignificant, and L2 proficiency did not contribute significantly to the performances of the Flanker task in all three conditions and conflict effect (*p*s>.05).

Therefore, in terms of the current data analyses, L2 proficiency played a limited role in distinguishing the ability of conflict monitoring and inhibition in cognitive control (as tested in the Flanker).

5.4.3 Number Stroop Task

Table 7 lists the detailed descriptive data of the two groups' performances in the Number Stroop task.

Table 7. Mean reaction times, Number Stroop conflict, and standard deviations in the Number Stroop task between groups differing in L2.

	Higher L2 group n=41		*Lower L2 group n=60*		*p value*
	M	*SD*	*M*	*SD*	*(t-test)*
Number Stroop neutral	735.9	107.9	727.2	84.2	.651
Number Stroop incongruent	732.7	98.3	732.4	88.5	.988
Number Stroop congruent	693.7	95.9	695.2	71.7	.928
Number Stroop conflict*	39.0	63.2	37.2	53.5	.623

Note. * Number Stroop conflict refers to the RT difference between incongruent and congruent conditions.

In this task, we analyzed the same indicators: global RTs in each condition and conflict effect, as we did in the Flanker task. Global RTs reflect the ability to monitor the potential conflict and conflict effect reflects the ability to inhibit an interfering (i.e., dominant) information/ response in favor of an unusual one. But compared with the Flanker task, the Number Stroop requires higher cognitive load. We expect that the higher L2 proficiency group will perform better/faster in this task than the lower L2 proficiency group. Four participants from the two groups were excluded because of false operations.

Similarly, we conducted repeated measures analysis of variance with language group (higher L2 group, lower L2 group) as between subject variable and condition (congruent, neutral, and incongruent) as within subject variables to compare the differences in the performance of the Number Stroop task between the two groups that differed in L2 proficiency.

The analysis of repeated measures showed that in the Number Stroop task performance, the main effect of condition was significant, F (2, 198) =25.988; p<.001; η^2=.208. Planned comparisons showed that participants did not respond more quickly in the neutral condition (730.72 ms) than in the incongruent condition (732.50 ms) (p=.876), but participants responded more quickly in the congruent condition (694.62 ms) than in the neutral (730.72 ms) and incongruent conditions (732.50 ms) (ps<.001), reflecting a significant Stroop conflict effect (RT difference between congruent and incongruent condition). However, the analysis revealed no main effect of participant group F (1, 99) =.022, p=.883, and the interaction between participant group and Number Stroop condition was not significant F (2, 198) =.410, p=.664, reflecting that there were no group differences in the speed and efficiency in performing the three conditions of the Number Stroop task. Furthermore, independent sample t-test analysis showed that there was no difference in terms of Number Stroop conflict (RTs difference between congruent and incongruent condition) between groups (p=.623), reflecting that the two groups did not differ in conflict resolution when congruent and incongruent trials were mixed.

Likewise, in order to further clarify the role of L2 proficiency in the Number Stroop task performance, we conducted multiple regression analysis by entering L2 proficiency, age, L2 history, and L2 exposure as independent variables. The results showed that the multiple regression models (Fs<1) were nonsignificant, and L2 proficiency did not contribute significantly to the performances of the Number Stroop task in all three conditions and conflict effect (ps>.05).

Therefore, the results in the Number Stroop task echoed that of the Flanker task. Between the two young-adult Chinese-English bilingual groups who differed in L2 proficiency, there were no group differences in performing the Number Stroop task, either in the trial type speed or the conflict effect. This means that the two groups had no significant differences in the aspects of conflict monitoring or inhibition in cognitive control, even though there was significant difference between them in L2 proficiency. As mentioned above, compared with the Flanker task, the Number Stroop task has a relatively higher cognitive load, but the two bilingual groups still did not distinguish in the abilities of conflict monitoring and inhibition in cognitive control. In contrast, the results from the two tasks consistently indicate that L2 proficiency alone may not play a significant role in enhancing bilinguals' cognitive control, specifically in the aspects of conflict monitoring and inhibition.

However, as cognitive control is composed of different subcomponents, the results still do not rule out a possibility that the higher L2 proficiency group may be superior to the lower L2 proficiency group in the aspect of mental set shifting, which is measured by the WCST task.

5.4.4 WCST

The WCST task was used to detect participants' mental set shifting: the ability to switch their mental set and their flexibility to infer the sorting rule or the ability to shift back and forth between multiple tasks, operations, or mental sets (Miyake et al., 2000; Yudes et al., 2011). In this task, we report global performance (RTs, completed categories, overall errors) and different types of errors (perseverative errors, previous category errors) as dependent variables to compare performance differences in mental set shifting between the two groups (Barceló & Knight, 2002). The means and standard deviations of RTs, completed categories, overall errors, perseverative errors, and previous category errors between the two groups are presented in Table 8. One participant was excluded due to false operations.

Independent sample *t*-test analysis of global RTs showed that there was no significant difference between the groups ($p=.132$), which means that the two groups responded equally quickly in executing the WCST task.

The total number of completed categories ranged from "0" to "19". "0" means the participant was not able to complete at least 5 consecutive correct responses to any of the categories. "19" means the participant successfully completed all the categories. The results of independent sample *t*-test on the number of completed categories showed that there was no significant difference between the two groups (p=.673). In addition, results from an independent sample t-test with the overall errors as the dependent variable revealed no significant difference between the two groups (p=.369).

Table 8. Mean reaction times and standard deviations of global performances and types of errors in the WCST between groups differing in L2.

	Higher L2 group n=43		*Lower L2 group n=61*		*p value*
	M	*SD*	*M*	*SD*	*(t-test)*
Global RTs	1555.5	526.3	1413.7	425.2	.132
Completed Categories	9.2	3.4	8.9	3.5	.673
Overall errors	57.7	14.1	60.4	15.5	.369
Perseverative errors	37.3	15.3	39.7	17.2	.459
Previous category errors	19.9	13.1	22.2	16.1	.444

According to Heaton et al. (1993), errors can be distinguished between perseverative and non-perseverative errors. Perseverative errors are failures to change the mental rule after receiving negative feedback so that the person continues sorting the cards according to the previous-category dimension despite feedback indicating that the response is wrong (Heaton et al., 1993; Yudes et al., 2011). Moreover, the errors can be further categorized into two types: perseverations to the immediately preceding category and perseverations to a different category. Previous category perseverations reflect a lack of flexibility in changing the mental set to a new rule, while different category perseverations reflect the understanding that the previous rule is no longer correct but there is an unsuccessful attempt to infer a new rule (Hartman et al., 2003; Yudes et al., 2011).

An independent sample *t*-test analysis was conducted to examine the distribution of these types of errors. The *t*-test results of perseverative errors showed no significant differences between the two groups (p=.459). The *t*-test performed on the number of previous-category errors revealed a null effect of group (p=.444).

Again, in order to further clarify the role of L2 proficiency in the WCST task performance, we conducted multiple regression analysis by entering L2 proficiency, age, L2 history, L2 exposure, and L2 using as independent variables. The results showed that the multiple regression models (Fs<1 for RTs, completed categories, overall errors, and perseverative errors; F (4, 99) =1.123 for previous category errors) were nonsignificant, and L2 proficiency did not contribute significantly to the performances of the WCST task (ps>.05).

To summarize, the results of dependent variables of the global RTs, completed categories, overall errors, perseverative errors, and previous category errors consistently show that there are no performance differences in the task WCST between the two bilingual groups, who differed significantly in L2 proficiency. Additional regression analyses suggest that L2 proficiency does not contribute significantly to the enhancement of cognitive control in mental set shifting. Combined with the results from the Flanker task and the Number Stroop task, we now reiterate the result contrasts from all the three tasks, for a better view of the role of L2 proficiency in bilingual advantage. The higher L2 group and the lower L2 group had homogeneous demographic, intellectual and social economic background, and were matched on L2 background including L2 history and L2 exposure but differed in L2 proficiency (both in self-rated and objective measures). Therefore, if there were any differences between the two groups in the Flanker task, the Number Stroop task, or the WCST task performances, we would attribute them to the differences of L2 language proficiency. However, the ANOVA and regression results of these tasks reveal that the role of L2 proficiency is limited under some circumstances and L2 proficiency alone does not contribute significantly to the enhancement of cognitive control among young adult Chinese-English bilinguals, specifically, in the aspects of inhibition, conflict monitoring, and mental set shifting.

5.5 Discussion

The current experiment examines the relationship between L2 proficiency and three aspects of cognitive control: conflict monitoring, inhibition, and mental set shifting, by administering the Flanker task, the Number Stroop task, and the WCST task between two bilingual groups differing in L2 proficiency. Between the two bilingual groups that we tested, there is no bilingual advantage for the higher L2 proficiency group in all the three tasks. Compared with the lower L2 proficiency group, the higher L2 proficiency group does not show faster RTs or smaller conflict effect in the Flanker task and the Number Stroop task, or better performance in the WCST task, while other factors such as IQ, L2 history and L2 exposure are matched. Further regression analyses results in the current experiment indicate that L2 proficiency is not strongly or directly related to bilingual advantage in the three aspects of cognitive control we just tested.

These results are not consistent to previous reports of a language proficiency (particularly L2) effect on bilingual advantage. A few previous studies indicate that language proficiency modulates cognitive control in bilinguals (e.g., Abutalebi et al., 2013; Iluz-Cohen & Armon-Lotem, 2013; Marian et al., 2013). Young adult bilinguals with higher L2 proficiency react faster than lower L2 proficiency bilinguals in target detection tasks (Mishra et al., 2012). Language proficiency has been reported significantly associated with cognitive control in Stroop task (Singh & Mishra, 2013) or attention network task (Videsott et al., 2012).

The absence of performance differences in the three cognitive control tasks between the two bilingual groups may be attributed to some influential factors.

First of all, similarly discussed in Chapter Four, age may be an important factor modulating the effect of bilingual advantage. In the current experiment, the participants are young adults in their early twenties. They are at the peak of their cognitive development, which means that they perform executive control tasks at very high efficiency. If this is true, the effect of bilingualism may provides little boost (Bialystok et al., 2009). Provided that other conditions are equal, a comparison between older adult or child bilingual groups who differ in L2 proficiency is more likely to produce an observable effect of bilingual advantage.

Secondly, task demand may also modulate the effect of bilingual advantage. Bilinguals may show an advantage relative to monolinguals only in high cognitive demand tasks (Costa et al., 2009). This condition may also extend to the case between bilinguals of different L2 proficiency degrees. But we shall be cautious about the speculation because in the current experiment although different tasks differing in cognitive demand are adopted (as the Flanker task and the Number Stroop task), the effect is still absent.

Thirdly, more importantly, we operationally classify the two bilingual groups into higher and lower L2 proficiency groups by statistical means, but in the field there is no standardized method for determining the degree of bilingualism (Prior & Gollan, 2011), causing the role of language proficiency in bilingual cognitive control advantage to remain ambiguous and indirect. Language proficiency does not tell us exactly to what extent bilinguals of different proficiency will differ in cognitive control. As in the current experiment, the two Chinese-English bilingual groups differ statistically in L2 proficiency, but practically the magnitude perhaps is not great enough (self-rating: 23.2 vs. 21.0; verbal fluency: 24.4 vs. 21.4). There is still a high possibility that if the L2 proficiency gap between the two bilingual groups had been greater, the effect would have emerged. We still stand by the view that L2 proficiency may contribute to bilingual cognitive control advantage in some limited or indirect ways.

Finally, language proficiency alone does not discriminate how differently bilinguals are using their languages. The specific bilingual language use experience in specific language context (Green & Abutalebi, 2013) must be very important factor determining bilingual advantage in specific aspects of cognitive control. Furthermore, there may be an interaction between language proficiency and language use, so the multiple related dimensions of bilingual language use experience need to be considered in assessments of bilingual advantage (Luk & Bialystok, 2013). In future research, we need to clarify and single out these factors. For example, we can compare bilinguals who have a particular language use experience with those who do not have such experience, with language proficiency manipulated at the same time.

5.6 Conclusion

In conclusion, by adopting the Flanker task, the Number Stroop task, and the WCST, the overall results in *Experiment Two* fail to capture cognitive control differences between two young adult unbalanced Chinese-English bilingual groups, who differ significantly in L2 proficiency. These results indicate that bilingual language proficiency (i.e. L2) alone does not necessarily bring about cognitive control differences among bilinguals, particularly in the aspects of inhibition, conflict monitoring, and mental set shifting. The complexity of language proficiency construct may lie in various degrees of bilingualism and in possible interactions between language proficiency and language use. Genuine enhancement of cognitive control abilities may come with greater differences in L2 proficiency or with some significant variables involved in bilingualism, such as language use experiences and their respective relationship with specific aspects of cognitive control. Therefore, in future studies, classifying different types of bilingualism and isolating confounding factors such as language use (e.g., language switching) from language proficiency may be helpful to identify the relationship between specific features of bilingualism and specific aspects of cognitive control among bilinguals. We will address these questions in the following two chapters.

Chapter 6: Experiment Three – Language Interpreting Experience and Cognitive Control[8]

6.1 Introduction

The results of *Experiment Two* reveal that L2 proficiency does not significantly contribute to cognitive control differences in the three aspects that have been tested: inhibition, conflict monitoring, and mental set shifting. Aside from possible factors such as participants' age, task demand, and the construct of proficiency etc., which may have caused the null effect of bilingual advantage, it is suggested that at least L2 proficiency is not a strong or sensitive factor directly affecting cognitive control and it may have an interaction between one important variable – specific language use experiences. The current experiment investigates this issue by taking language interpreting as one such example. It is to answer *Research Question 3* in the current doctoral research: *Does language interpreting experience contribute to cognitive control differences among young-adult bilinguals?*

6.2 Specific Background

In previous literature, little empirical work has been done for general cognitive control differences between different bilingual groups or for

8 The main part of this study has been published in the *Journal of Cognitive Psychology* as Yanping Dong & Zhilong Xie (2014). Contributions of second language proficiency and interpreting experience to cognitive control differences among young adult bilinguals. *Journal of Cognitive Psychology*, 26(5), 506–519. doi:10.1080/20445911.2014.924951.

reasons underlying these differences. Generally speaking, factors that are able to explain cognitive control differences between different bilingual groups are most probably factors that are able to explain cognitive control differences between bilinguals and monolinguals. It is still reasonable that language proficiency (particularly L2 proficiency for unbalanced bilinguals) somehow contributes to bilingual advantage in cognitive control, since proficiency is the core essence of bilingualism. Although no cognitive control differences are found between the L2 proficiency differing bilingual groups in **Experiment Two**, it is still very likely that bilinguals' cognitive control enhancement (if any) is somehow related to their L2 proficiency (Videsott et al., 2012; Tse & Altarriba, 2012; Singh & Mishra, 2012; 2013; Iluz-Cohen & Armon-Lotem, 2013). However, the problem may lie in, very importantly, that language proficiency, as a complex construct (Hulstijn, 2012), cannot reveal what degrees of proficiency bilinguals should acquire in order to achieve qualitatively better cognitive control. Furthermore, as bilinguals' language proficiency increases, other confounding factors (such as more language switching and language using in a particular pattern) may obscure the effect. Therefore, it is necessary to isolate the confounding factors from language proficiency so as to find out specific aspects of bilingualism that may have caused bilingual advantage in cognitive control.

If language proficiency is manipulated, the most probable potentially confounding factor among bilinguals is their particular language use experience. Bilinguals may vary in how they use their languages and in how they use the languages in different community contexts (Green, 2011; Prior & Gollan, 2011). According to Green (2011), the community context in which bilingual speakers typically use their two languages (the behavioral ecology of bilingual speakers) should be adequately considered in the study of bilingual advantage. More recently, the adaptive control hypothesis (Green & Abutalebi, 2013) proposes that language control processes themselves adapt to the recurrent demands placed on them by the interactional context. Adapting a control process means changing a parameter or parameters about the way it works (its neural capacity or efficiency) or the way it works in concert, or in cascade, with other control processes (e.g., its connectedness). Therefore, different contexts (such as single or dual language context or intense language switching context) that require different cognitive demands will very likely lead to varied cognitive control adaptations.

One such typical example of interactional contexts is language interpreting, which involves intensive and intentional language switching practice between the two languages. A few previous studies have found some relationship between how frequently bilinguals switch their two languages in their daily life and their cognitive control abilities (Prior & Gollan, 2011; Rodriguez-Fornells, Kramer, Lorenzo-Seva, Festman, & Munte, 2011; Soveri, Rodriguez-Fornells, & Laine, 2011). In the context of language interpreting, it involves more intensive practice of language switching and therefore provides a good context to study bilingual control (De Groot & Christoffels, 2006). There have been studies indicating that compared to reading in the monolingual mode, the task of interpreting requires more activation of both languages while comprehending the source language (Dong & Lin, 2013; Yudes, Macizo, Morales, & Bajo, 2012), and that interpreters have to put great effort into coordinating both comprehension and production in the process of interpreting, especially in simultaneous interpreting[9] (Padilla, Bajo, & Macizo, 2005; Yudes, Macizo, & Bajo, 2012). These particular features inherent in the task of interpreting pose a special demand on language control to monitor, coordinate and separate the two languages during comprehension and production while continuously switching between them (Ibanez, Macizo, & Bajo, 2010). Interpreting training with this higher demand may thus enhance the efficiency of language control and eventually transfers to non-verbal cognitive control. Yudes, Macizo, and Bajo (2011) found that professional simultaneous

9 The two typical modes of interpreting are consecutive interpreting, in which the interpreter immediately begins the interpretation of a message after the speaker has stopped speaking, and simultaneous interpreting, in which the interpreter renders the interpretation while still receiving the source utterance. Apparently, the latter is cognitively more demanding, since the interpreter has to split his or her attention and exercise a tighter control of the whole process so that comprehension and production are well coordinated. Another form of intensive language switching experience is (written) translation. Since the task of translation generally does not require immediate rendition, it does not pose as much demand on language control as interpreting. And yet, the three forms of language switching experience all involve basically the same switching process, intensive switching between the two languages.

interpreters outperform control bilinguals and monolinguals in the cognitive control function of mental flexibility. In their study, a Simon task (which tested inhibition) and a WCST task (which tested shifting) were adopted. The results showed that professional interpreters did not perform differently from control bilinguals and monolinguals in the Simon task, but outperformed bilinguals and monolinguals on the WCST task, which suggests that experience in interpreting is more associated with cognitive flexibility (mental set shifting) in cognitive control. Therefore, investigating the relationship between language interpreting and cognitive control enhancement can help us find out the specific origins of bilingual advantage.

Based on previous discussions, the current experiment (**Experiment Three**) intends to investigate whether and how language interpreting experience contributes to cognitive control differences among young adult bilinguals, with L2 proficiency isolated from language interpreting experience. Our research rationale is: 1) if language interpreting experience plays a crucial role, bilinguals with or without such experience may perform differently in cognitive control tasks when other factors are controlled; 2) if language interpreting experience contributes to cognitive control, different length of interpreting training may also result in variations of cognitive control enhancement.

To find an answer for the question, we need to include: firstly, bilingual group(s) with interpreting experience and control bilingual group(s) without such experience; secondly, interpreting group with longer time of training experience and interpreting group with shorter time of training experience; thirdly, control bilingual groups differing in L2 proficiency. By comparing bilingual groups who have interpreting experience and control bilingual groups without such experience, we can find out whether such experience contributes to cognitive control differences among the bilinguals. By comparing interpreting groups who have different length of training, we can find out to what degree such training is effective in enhancing cognitive control. By including bilingual groups differing in L2 proficiency, we can manipulate the role of L2 proficiency and match L2 proficiency among those comparable bilingual groups.

Therefore, there are four groups of unbalanced Chinese-English bilinguals who differ in language interpreting experience and L2 proficiency (see the participants section for details) in the current experiment (**Experiment Three**). For consistency, all the participant groups were compared in terms of their performance on the same tasks adopted in Experiment One and Experiment Two: the Flanker task, the Number Stroop task, and the Wisconsin Card Sorting Test (WCST). As in Experiment One and Experiment Two, the Flanker task and the Number Stroop task are designed to test participants' conflict monitoring and inhibition, and the WCST is designed to measure participants' mental set shifting.

6.3 Method

6.3.1 Participants

One hundred and fifty-four Chinese-English right-handed young adult bilinguals (14 males/140 females) from a university in China, with a mean age of 21.58 years (SD=1.545), participated in this experiment for either financial compensation or course credit. All of them reported normal or corrected-to-normal vision and had no speech or hearing disorders. They gave informed consent, and their rights were protected in accordance with the ethical standards of the university's Academic Board.

There were four bilingual groups of participants: two with language interpreting experience, coded hereafter as Interpreting-1 and Interpreting-2, and two without language interpreting experience, coded as Noninterpreting-1 and Noninterpreting-2. The Interpreting groups were undergraduate or graduate students specializing in translation and interpreting studies in the university, with Interpreting-1 having received interpreting training for one year (tests taken at the end of third-year undergraduate studies), and Interpreting-2 for three years (tests taken at the end of first-year graduate studies). The Noninterpreting groups (Noninterpreting-1, Noninterpretint-2), as controls for the interpreting participants, were students majoring in general

English (English language and culture) who had received no formal training on language interpreting but differed in L2 proficiency before participating in this study. We included the *higher L2 proficiency group* from Experiment Two as the higher L2 proficiency bilingual group in the current experiment (as Noninterpreting-2) in order to match L2 proficiency with one of the interpreting groups.

The Interpreting groups took special courses, such as consecutive interpreting, translation[10], conference interpreting, interpreting workshops, etc., which could be classified as language switch training (half interpreting, half written translation). There were four such courses for each semester of about 18 weeks (two semesters in a year), with each course taking 80 minutes per session each week. After-class practice was generally required, amounting to about 8–16 hours each week. When Interpreting-1 participated in our study, they had taken eight such courses, amounting to 192 hours of class time in total. The class time for the group of Interpreting-2 was triple that of Interpreting-1.

All participants' previous experience with English (L2) was homogeneous in that they had started learning English as a foreign language (in the classroom) around age 10, in order to qualify for college enrollment. This suggests that the participants were unbalanced bilinguals who had few L2 communication needs in their everyday life (with English mostly used in classes of English, or when watching English videos or reading English books outside the classroom). To assess language proficiency (same as in Experiment 1), we required the participants to complete a composite questionnaire with questions tapping participants' language background, including self-rated language proficiency (Marian et al., 2007), and to perform an English (L2) verbal fluency test as an objective measurement. In the verbal fluency test, participants were required to produce as many words as possible according to the category presented (jobs, sports, animals) in 60 seconds. Category fluency is reported to be strongly indicative of

10 The current paper does not try to isolate the interpreting experience from that of translation, since interpreting and translation basically involve the same language switching process, and students receiving interpreting training generally receive translation training at the same time, although the reverse is not necessarily true.

vocabulary size (Bialystok et al., 2009). Table 9 is a summary of the participants' characteristics[11].

Table 9. Characteristics of participants groups: Noninterpreting-1, Noninterpreting-2, Interpreting-1, and Interpreting-2.

	Noninter-preting-1	*Noninter-preting-2*	*Interpreting-1*	*Interpreting-2*
	n=45	*n=43*	*n=46*	*n=20*
Age (years)	20.5^{a} (0.8)	22.4^{b} (1.8)	21.1^{c} (0.9)	23.3^{d} (1.2)
Learning History (years)	10.5^{a} (0.8)	12.4^{b} (1.7)	11.1^{c} (0.9)	13.3^{d} (1.2)
English Proficiency (0–40)	21.5^{a} (2.7)	23.2^{b} (4.5)	22.9^{b} (3.4)	29.8^{c} (3.3)
English Verbal Fluency	19.4^{a} (3.7)	24.4^{b} (4.2)	24.9^{b} (4.0)	30.5^{c} (5.0)
English exposure (%)	47.8 (21.5)	43.3 (17.7)	41.5 (16.2)	48.3 (16.6)
English use (%)	20.3^{a} (6.0)	21.3^{a} (5.7)	21.9^{a} (6.9)	29.3^{b} (7.0)
Interpreting Training (years)	0.0	0.0	1.0	3.0

Note. Means in the same row with different superscript letters differ from each other significantly at $p<.01$ or $p<.05$. The age difference is not practically significant since all were young adult bilinguals.

11 We did not assess participants' social economic status (SES) because they were not so much relevant to our participants in the present experiment. Although Hook et al. (2013) suggested an association between SES and cognitive control, this association is mostly based on child bilinguals (but see Prior & Gollan, 2011). Furthermore, the participants in the present experiment came from similar family and educational background. Thus we assumed that there was no systematic SES bias across the groups. As for IQ, as we had already tested in Experiment One and Experiment Two, there were no significant group differences. Moreover, since our participants were admitted to the same university after taking the same college entrance examination, it is unlikely that there were systematic IQ differences among the different participant groups. In addition, some previous studies show that working memory updating is highly correlated with intelligence measures, but other aspects such as inhibiting and mental set shifting tested in the present study are not (Friedman et al., 2006; Toplak et al., 2010).

As can be seen, the four groups differed in L2 proficiency at three levels[12]. Interpreting-2 had the highest English proficiency, which differed from the other groups ($ps<.001$); Interpreting-1 and Noninterpreting-2 were matched in L2 proficiency ($p=.608$); Noninterpreting-1 had the lowest language proficiency ($ps<.001$). At the same time, all the groups had the same percentage of English (L2) exposure (Chinese and English equal 100 percent) ($ps>.05$). However, Interpreting-2 had the highest percentage of English (L2) use ($ps<.001$), whereas Interpreting-1, Noninterpreting-2, and Noninterpreting-1 did not differ ($ps>.05$). There were statistically significant age differences across all the four groups. However, the factor of age difference was ignored in our analysis because all the participants could be categorized as young adult bilinguals (20.5–23.3 years old) and were in their prime of cognitive control abilities.

6.3.2 Materials and Procedure

The experiment lasted for about 1.5 hours. All the participants were firstly required to finish the background questionnaire as mentioned above and secondly required to complete the three cognitive control tasks measuring inhibition, conflict monitoring, and mental set shifting.

Cognitive Control Tasks

The same three computerized tasks (the Flanker task, the Number Stroop task, and the Wisconsin Card Sorting Task) from Experiment One were used to tap into participants' cognitive control on inhibition, conflict monitoring, and mental set shifting.

12 Only English proficiency was assessed. This is based on our presumption that our participants, who had passed a college entrance examination and were regular college students majoring in English or interpreting, must have concurrently maintained a high proficiency in their native language – Mandarin Chinese. We believe that there was no significant difference in their L1 proficiency (although there might be variations) due to the homogeneity of their educational background.

6.4 Result

6.4.1 Data Trimming

The final data set was created in the following ways: In the Flanker task and the Number Stroop task, data from erroneous responses were first excluded. We then calculated the mean reaction time (RT), and the standard deviation (SD) of each subject in each condition, and eliminated trials that were over 3 SDs above the mean (with a final data loss of 1.87% of all trials). In the WCST task, we first calculated the mean RT for each of the subjects in each condition, and excluded trials that fell 3 SDs above or below the mean (1.32% of all trials). We then counted the characteristic indexes of the WSCT task for each participant, including completed categories, overall errors and types of errors.

6.4.2 Flanker Task

Table 10 is a summary of the descriptive data for the Flanker task. The measured dependent variables were the overall response times in each condition and the Flanker conflict. To determine whether the bilingual groups of higher proficiency would complete the task more efficiently than the bilingual groups of lower proficiency and whether the language interpreting groups would outperform the non-interpreting groups, we conducted a repeated measures analysis of variance (ANOVA), with participant groups (Interpreting-1, Noninterpreting-1, Interpreting-2, Noninterpreting-2) as a between-subject variable and condition (neutral, incongruent, congruent) as the within-subject variable.

Table 10. Means (standard deviations) of reaction times and Flanker conflict in the Flanker task across interpreting and control groups.

	Noninter-preting-1	*Noninter-preting-2*	*Interpreting-1*	*Interpreting-2*
	n=45	*n=43*	*n=46*	*n=20*
Flanker neutral	543.1 (103.1)	536.0 (91.3)	532.7 (75.6)	517.5 (89.8)
Flanker incongruent	583.1 (110.6)	578.3 (87.1)	569.2 (83.0)	548.2 (66.6)
Flanker congruent	527.8 (119.4)	516.4 (80.6)	518.4 (73.1)	497.0 (85.8)
Flanker conflict*	55.3 (36.0)	61.9 (49.5)	50.8 (32.5)	51.2 (35.3)

Note. *Flanker conflict refers to the RT difference between incongruent and congruent conditions.

The analysis revealed a significant main effect of trial condition F (2, 300) =151.246, $p<.001$, $\eta^2=.502$. Pairwise comparisons showed that participants responded more quickly in the congruent condition (517.80 ms) than in the neutral (534.68 ms) and incongruent conditions (573.07 ms) ($ps<.001$), and participants responded more quickly in the neutral condition (534.68 ms) than in the incongruent condition (573.07 ms) ($p<.001$), reflecting a significant Flanker effect (difference between congruent and incongruent condition). However, the analysis revealed no main effect of participant group F (3,150) =.553, $p=.647$, and the interaction between participant group and Flanker condition was not significant F (6,300) =.496, $p=.811$, reflecting that there were no group differences in the speed and efficiency in performing the three conditions of the Flanker task. Moreover, an ANOVA analysis showed that there were no group differences in terms of Flanker conflict (RTs difference between congruent and incongruent condition) across groups F (3,150) =.641, $p=.590$, reflecting that the four groups did not differ in conflict resolution when congruent and incongruent trials were mixed. Further post-hoc tests showed that there were no group differences between any groups among the four on each of the condition (neutral, incongruent, congruent) and on conflict effect.

6.4.3 Number Stroop Task

Table 11 is a summary of the descriptive data for the Number Stroop task. Three participants were excluded because of false operations. The measured dependent variables were the overall response times in each condition and the Number Stroop conflict. To determine whether the bilingual groups of higher proficiency would complete the task more efficiently than the bilingual groups of lower proficiency and whether the language interpreting groups would outperform the non-interpreting groups, we conducted a repeated measures analysis of variance with participant groups (Interpreting-1, Noninterpreting-1, Interpreting-2, Noninterpreting-2) as a between-subject variable and condition (neutral, incongruent, congruent) as the within-subject variable.

The analysis revealed a significant main effect of trial condition $F(2, 294) = 44.099, p < .001, \eta^2 = .231$. Pairwise comparisons showed that participants did not respond more quickly in the neutral condition (731.17 ms) than in the incongruent condition (730.59 ms) ($p = .884$), but participants responded more quickly in the congruent condition (692.90 ms) than in the neutral (731.17 ms) and incongruent conditions (730.59 ms) ($ps < .001$), reflecting a significant Number Stroop effect (difference between congruent and incongruent condition). However, the analysis revealed no main effect of participant group $F(3,147) = 1.167, p = .325$, and the interaction between participant group and Flanker condition was not significant $F(6, 294) = .172, p = .984$, reflecting that there were no group differences in the speed and efficiency in performing the three conditions of the Number Stroop task. Moreover, an ANOVA analysis showed that there were no group differences in terms of Number Stroop conflict (RTs difference between congruent and incongruent condition) across groups $F(3,146) = .181, p = .909$, reflecting that the four groups did not differ in conflict resolution when congruent and incongruent trials were mixed. Post-hoc tests showed that there were no group differences between any groups among the four on each of the condition (neutral, incongruent, congruent) and on conflict effect.

Table 11. Means (standard deviations) of reaction times and Stroop conflict in the Number Stroop task across interpreting and control groups.

	Noninter-preting-1	*Noninter-preting-2*	*Interpret-ing-1*	*Interpret-ing-2*
	n=44	*n=41*	*n=46*	*n=20*
Number Stroop neutral	747.4 (78.8)	735.9 (107.9)	716.0 (86.2)	720.7 (97.5)
Number Stroop incongruent	746.6 (92.3)	732.7 (98.3)	718.4 (75.7)	719.4 (96.8)
Number Stroop congruent	711.0 (67.4)	693.7 (95.9)	682.6 (77.2)	675.2 (81.0)
Number Stroop conflict*	35.6 (57.6)	39.0 (63.2)	35.8 (43.2)	44.2 (50.9)

Note. * Number Stroop conflict refers to the RT difference between incongruent and congruent conditions.

The four groups differed both in language interpreting experience and L2 proficiency. As can be seen in Table 9, Interpreting-2 had the highest L2 proficiency and also used the L2 the most (which differed from the other groups with *ps* $< .001$); Interpreting-1 and Noninterpreting-2 were homogeneous in L2 proficiency with $p = .608$; Noninterpreting-1 had the lowest L2 proficiency (*ps* $< .001$). However, there were no differences across groups, either in speed, or in conflict resolution, on the Flanker task and the Number Stroop task. We further ran analyses comparing only 2 levels, namely interpreting vs. non-interpreting, with L2 proficiency (verbal fluency scores) as a covariate. The two task results neither showed any significant effect of interpreting experience on overall reaction times of the three trial types, nor on the task conflict (Flanker neutral: $F < 1, p = .804$; Flanker incongruent: $F < 1, p = .816$; Flanker congruent: $F < 1, p = .948$; Flanker conflict: $F < 1, p = .530$; Number Stroop neutral: $F<1, p=.719$; Number Stroop incongruent: $F<1$, $p=.676$; Number Stroop congruent: $F<1$, $p=.977$; Number Stroop conflict: $F<1, p=.430$). In short, both the Flanker task and the Number Stroop task results indicate that, in terms of reaction times and conflict resolution, neither language interpreting experience nor L2 proficiency plays a significant role in distinguishing the ability of inhibition and conflict monitoring in cognitive control across the bilingual groups.

6.4.4 WCST

Global performance (RTs, completed categories, overall errors) and different types of errors (perseverative errors, previous category errors) are reported as dependent variables to compare performance differences in mental flexibility (Barceló & Knight, 2002) across the groups. Table 12 presents the means and standard deviations of RTs, completed categories, overall errors, perseverative errors, and previous category errors across groups.

Table 12. Means (standard deviations) of reaction times, completed categories, errors etc. in the WCST across interpreting and control groups.

	Noninterpreting-1	*Noninterpreting-2*	*Interpreting-1*	*Interpreting-2*
	n=45	*n*=43	*n*=46	*n*=20
Global RTs	1425.8 (433.2)	1555.5 (526.3)	1449.5(490.2)	1503.5(438.5)
Completed Categories	9.0^{a} (3.5)	9.2^{a} (3.4)	11.0^{b} (3.3)	12.8^{c} (3.4)
Overall errors	60.1^{a} (14.9)	57.7^{a} (14.1)	47.8^{b} (11.2)	43.0^{b} (12.7)
Perseverative errors	39.8^{a} (17.0)	37.3^{a} (15.3)	26.2^{b} (10.7)	21.9^{b} (14.3)
Previous category errors	22.0^{a} (15.9)	19.9^{a} (13.1)	11.8^{b} (8.0)	8.2^{b} (8.1)

Note. Means in the same row with different superscript letters differ from each other significantly at $p<.01$ or $p<.05$.

Global performances. The ANOVA analysis of *global RTs* showed that there were no significant differences across the groups, $F(3, 150) = .628$, $p = .598$. The total number of categories ranged from 0 (which means the participant was unable to complete at least 5 consecutive correct responses to any of the categories) to 19 (which means the participant successfully completed all the categories). The results of ANOVA on the number of *completed categories* showed that there were significant differences across the groups, $F(3, 150) = 7.798, p < .001, \eta^2 = .135$. Post-hoc analyses showed that Interpreting-2 completed the highest number of categories compared to the two non-interpreting groups (Noninterpreting-1: $p < .001$; Noninterpreting-2: $p < .001$). Moreover, between the two interpreting groups, Interpreting-2, who had had a longer language interpreting experience, higher L2 proficiency and more L2 use, completed significantly more categories than Interpreting-1 (p = .048). In addition, Interpreting-1, similar to Interpreting-2, completed a higher number of categories compared to Noninterpreting-1 (p = .006) and Noninterpreting-2 (p = .013). However, there was no group difference between the two non-interpreting groups (p = .819), who differed in L2 proficiency. The ANOVA analysis on the *overall errors* revealed a significant difference across groups, F (3, 150) = 12.051, $p < .001$, $\eta^2 = .194$. Post-hoc multiple comparisons showed that both Interpreting-1 and Interpreting-2 made fewer errors than Noninterpreting-1 and Noninterpreting-2 (p = .001, $p < .001$ respectively). However, there was no group difference between the two interpreting groups (p = .179) or between the two non-interpreting groups (p = .395).

Types of errors. Heaton et al. (1993) distinguish between perseverative and non-perseverative errors. Perseverative errors represent failures to change the mental rule after receiving negative feedback, so that the test candidate continues sorting the cards according to the previous category dimension(s), despite feedback indicating that the response has been wrong (Heaton et al., 1993; Yudes et al., 2011). In addition, the errors can be further categorized into perseverations of the immediately preceding category and perseverations of a different category (Hartman et al., 2003; Yudes et al., 2011). Previous category perseverations reflect a lack of flexibility in changing the mental set to a new rule, while different category perseverations reflect the understanding that the previous rule is no longer correct, but there has been an unsuccessful attempt to infer a new rule. An ANOVA analysis was conducted to examine the distribution of these types of errors in each group. The ANOVA results of *perseverative errors* showed significant differences across the groups, F (3, 150) = 11.784, $p < .001$, $\eta^2 = .191$. Further post-hoc multiple comparisons indicated that the two interpreting groups made fewer perseverative errors than the two non-interpreting groups (ps < .001). However, there was no group difference between the two interpreting groups (p = .265), or between the two non-interpreting groups (p = .420). The ANOVA performed on the number of *previous-category errors* revealed a significant group effect, F (3, 150) = 9.527, $p < .001$, $\eta^2 = .160$, with post-hoc analyses indicating that Interpreting-2 made fewer previous category errors than the two non-interpreting groups (ps < .001), and that Interpreting-1 also made fewer such errors than the two non-interpreting groups ($p = .002$, $p < .001$ respectively). However, there was neither any difference between the two interpreting groups ($p = .269$), nor between the two non-interpreting groups ($p = .434$).

Further analysis. To provide further support for the role of interpreting experience in cognitive control, we divided Interpreting-1 into two subgroups: one with higher L2 proficiency (20 participants), and the other with lower L2 proficiency (26 participants), so that we had a group of participants who were different from Interpreting-2 in the years of interpreting training they had received, but at the same level of L2 proficiency (verbal fluency) (p=.131). The two interpreting groups (Interpreting-1-subgroup and Interpreting-2), comparable in L2 proficiency, were different in completed categories in WCST (p=.039), and the differences between the two groups in overall errors and previous-category errors were marginally significant (p=.077, p=.069 respectively), but without any group differences in overall reaction times and perseverative errors (see Table 13). In other words, while there were differences in some of the WCST indices between the two groups of participants with different years of interpreting training, the contrast between these two groups was not as sharp as the contrast between those who had received interpreting training and those who had not. This is robust support for the role of language interpreting experience in cognitive control enhancement, i.e. the mental set shifting measured in the WCST task.

However, this does not exclude the contribution of the factor of L2 use, since Interpreting-2 had also reported a higher percentage of L2 use (p=.011) while Interpreting-1 subgroup and Interpreting-2 were matched on L2 proficiency and L2 exposure (see Table 13). In order to further sort out which factor(s) may have contributed significantly to the mental set shifting advantage for the interpreter bilinguals, we conducted a stepwise multiple regression analysis. L2 proficiency (verbal fluency scores), L2 use, and L2 exposure were measured as continuous variables, while interpreting experience was classified into three levels with '0' representing no interpreting experience, '1' representing one year's interpreting training and '2' three years' interpreting training. The results showed that L2 proficiency, L2 exposure and L2 use did not significantly predict bilinguals' performances in the WCST task (Fs < 1, *ps* > .10), but interpreting experience did: completed categories, adjusted $R^2 = .125$, $F(1, 149) = 22.429$, $p < .001$; overall errors, adjusted $R^2 = .172$, $F(1, 149) = 32.071$, $p < .001$; preservative errors, adjusted $R^2 = .167$, $F(1, 149) = 31.018$, $p < .001$; and previous category errors, adjusted $R^2 = .140$, $F(1, 149) = 25.502$, $p < .001$.

Table 13. Characteristics of Interpreting-1 subgroup and Interpreting-2 and their performances in the WCST task.

	Interpreting-1 subgroup	*Interpreting-2*	*(t-test) p value*
	n=20	*n=20*	
English Verbal Fluency	28.65 (1.1)	30.45 (5.0)	.131
English exposure (%)	48.3 (16.6)	50.4 (15.8)	.677
English use (%)	22.8 (8.4)	29.3 (7.0)	.011
Global RTs	1345.5 (371.1)	1503.5 (438.5)	.226
Completed Categories	10.4 (3.9)	12.8 (3.4)	.039
Overall errors	50.1 (12.2)	43.0 (12.7)	.077
Perseverative errors	28.0 (10.6)	21.9 (14.3)	.130
Previous category errors	13.2 (9.0)	8.2 (8.1)	.069

Summary. To provide a clearer view for the role of interpreting experience, we now summarize the contrasts[13]. First, Interpreting-1 and Noninterpreting-2 were matched on L2 proficiency (both in self-rated and objective measures), L2 exposure and L2 use, but differed in language interpreting experience. The ANOVA results of the WCST revealed that Interpreting-1 performed significantly better than Noninterpreting-2 on completed categories, overall errors, perseverative errors, and previous category errors. Second, between the two Noninterpreting groups, who did not have any interpreting experience and who differed in L2 proficiency, there were no significant differences on any of the dependent

13 We noticed that there were significant age differences across all the four groups. However, the factor of age difference was ignored in our analysis because all the participants could be categorized as young adult bilinguals and were in their prime of cognitive control abilities. Moreover, even if this age difference played a significant role in our study, the results would be that the group of Interpreting-2 should be the slowest performers (since they were the oldest), which is obviously contradictory to our findings.

variables we examined (completed categories, overall errors, perseverative errors, and previous category errors). Third, between the two interpreting groups that differed in years of interpreting training, there were significant differences in some of the WCST indices when L2 proficiency was matched. Fourth, regression analysis revealed no effect for L2 proficiency (or L2 use or L2 exposure), but a significant effect for interpreting experience. To sum up, the WCST task results show that there are robust differences between groups differing in language interpreting experience, no matter L2 proficiency is matched or not.

6.5 Discussion

Our research question for the current experiment is how language interpreting experience contributes to cognitive control differences among young-adult bilinguals, with the role of L2 proficiency manipulated. The experimental results are consistent with those in Experiment Two, which reveal that for young-adult bilinguals, L2 proficiency fail to contribute to cognitive control differences either in inhibition, conflict monitoring, or in mental set shifting as measured respectively in the Flanker task, the Number Stroop task, and the WSCT task. However, language interpreting experience significantly contributes to cognitive control differences in mental set shifting but not in inhibition or conflict monitoring.

The failure to find the role of L2 proficiency in cognitive control advantages runs contrary to findings from a few previous studies with children (Iluz-Cohen & Armon-Lotem, 2013; Videsott et al., 2012), or young adults (Singh & Mishra, 2012, 2013; Tse & Altarriba, 2012). As in Experiment Two, this may be attributed to a few reasons. First, similar to Bialystok et al.'s (2009) explanation that bilingualism offers no further boost for young adults who are at the peak age of their cognitive capacities (Bialystok et al., 2008; Bialystok et al., 2005; Paap & Greenberg, 2013; Salvatierra & Rosselli, 2011), higher L2 proficiency may not always bring about more cognitive control advantages in young adults. Second, the presence or absence of cognitive control advantages may be related to task difficulty, such as to what extent the task demands one's attention (Costa et al., 2009). The current experiment results do not reveal any group differences in the Flanker task and the Number Stroop task although the two tasks differed in task difficulty, but in all, the tasks might be too easy for the young adults. Third, more importantly, L2 proficiency is a very complex construct, which is hard to measure and isolate from factors such as L2 use, L2 experience, etc. The improvement of L2 proficiency is probably accompanied by more L2 use, or more language switching experience (especially in a specific context). In addition, it is difficult to define how much language proficiency is needed before a cognitive control advantage shows up in behavioral measures. A larger language proficiency gap may be able to produce significant cognitive control differences among bilingual groups. Moreover, higher L2 proficiency may result in a more balanced use of the two languages, which in turn may lead to more significant cognitive control advantages (Zied et al., 2004). Apparently, though, the participants in the current experiment are unbalanced L2 learners.

More importantly, as for the role of language interpreting experience, we have found that bilinguals with language interpreting experience perform significantly better than bilinguals without such experience on the aspect of mental set shifting (as tested in the WCST), when L2 proficiency is manipulated. Even between the two proficiency-matched interpreting sub-groups, who had received interpreting training for different lengths of time (1 year and 3 years respectively), there are significant or marginal differences in the WCST indices (see Table 13). This result is consistent with that of Experiment One and with some previous findings that bilinguals outperform monolinguals in the task WCST, or similar task, since bilinguals have much experience of switching between two languages while monolinguals have none (Bialystok, 1999; Bialystok & Martin, 2004; Taler, Johns, Young, Sheppard, & Jones, 2013). The result is also consistent with Yudes et al. (2011), which find that professional interpreters outperform bilinguals and monolinguals in the WCST task.

Although the current result is similar to Yudes et al. (2011) in a number of respects, it also differs from it in certain ways. Yudes et al. (2011) aimed at exploring cognitive control processes in simultaneous interpreters, and thus compared how three groups of participants (simultaneous interpreters, bilinguals without simultaneous training and monolinguals) performed in the WCST and Simon tasks. In contrast, the current experiment aimed at exploring what role language interpreting experience may play in cognitive control variations among unbalanced bilinguals, and thus compared how bilinguals differing in interpreting experience performed in the WCST and the Flanker and the Number Stroop tasks. The first difference between the two is that, in Yudes et al. (2011), monolinguals were included, and language proficiency was controlled, while in the current experiment monolinguals were not included[14] and proficiency was manipulated. The second difference is that, in Yudes et al. (2011), a Simon task was used to capture response inhibition, whereas in the current experiment a Flanker task and a Number Stroop task were used to capture inhibition of a distracting stimulus and conflict monitoring. The third difference is that, in Yudes et al. (2011), the bilinguals were more or less balanced in the two languages, and the professional simultaneous interpreters had around 10.83 years of interpreting experience, while in the current experiment, the bilinguals were unbalanced, and the student interpreters had only had 1 or 3 years of interpreting training. Hence although the two studies are similar and yield similar results, they both contribute to the literature by manipulating vs. controlling L2 proficiency and exploring the role of different types of inhibitory control, as well as the role of different lengths of time in interpreting experience. The fact that the pattern of results is similar in the two studies provides further evidence for the general conclusion that language interpreting experience significantly contributes to cognitive control differences in mental set shifting, but not in inhibition or conflict monitoring. Particular contributions from the current experiment are findings for the comparison of different lengths of interpreting training time (one vs. three years), which again provides further support for the general conclusion.

The current experiment focuses on one of the most important aspects of bilingualism that are considered relevant to bilingual

14 Since the Noninterpreting-2 group in Experiment Three was the same bilingual group measured in Experiment One, we actually have already found that the bilinguals performed better than the monolinguals in the WCST.

advantage, that is, bilingual language use experience, or to be more specific, interpreting experience. L2 proficiency may be a factor that can enhance cognitive control abilities, although it is absent in the current experiment. But taking all the relevant results into consideration, it seems that, for young adult bilinguals, the specific experience of interpreting training is a more powerful factor in mental set shifting enhancement. There is evidence indicating that switching between languages increases pre-SMA/ACC (pre-Supplementary Motor Area/Anterior Cingulate Cortex) response, regardless of the proficiency differences of the two languages that bilinguals have acquired (Abutalebi et al., 2013). As to why language switching experience enhances cognitive control abilities, relevant research illustrates that language switching leads to the recruitment of brain regions of the left inferior frontal cortex, the caudate and the anterior cingulate among bilinguals (Garbin et al., 2011; Garbin et al., 2010), which overlap with the regions responsible for non-linguistic cognitive control. This overlap of brain regions has led researchers to speculate that the continuous employment of these regions in language switching strengthens the capability and increases the efficiency of related brain functions in nonlinguistic domains.

But then why is it that the student interpreter bilinguals do not outperform their non-interpreter counterparts regarding inhibition or conflict monitoring? According to Yudes et al. (2011), the experience in interpreting does not necessarily improve all the aspects of cognitive control because the nature of interpreting seems to be independent of the type of inhibition or monitoring required by tasks such as the Simon, the Stroop, or Flanker tasks. Interpreting may not require intense inhibition/conflict monitoring, since the two languages are kept active for comprehension and production, but the mental flexibility to switch from one language to another is crucial (Ibanez et al., 2010; Yudes et al., 2011).

If all confounding factors are controlled, a test of the role of potential factors in cognitive control differences *among* young adult bilinguals is a more delicate test of bilingual advantages than a direct comparison between bilinguals and monolinguals. If significant effects for these potential factors can be found among young adult bilinguals, these effects are most likely to appear in the same tests when bilinguals and monolinguals are compared, although the *absence* of such effects among bilinguals does not necessarily mean an absence of bilingual advantage when bilinguals and monolinguals are compared. Since the current experiment is interested in identifying how interpreting experience, with L2 proficiency manipulated, contributes to cognitive control differences among young adult bilinguals, we can not conclude that L2 proficiency is not related to cognitive control advantages, but, on the other hand, we can make the conclusion that participants' interpreting experience is an important factor in cognitive control enhancement (in mental set shifting). The current experiment therefore represents part of the effort to explore whether and how specific bilingual language use experience affects general domain cognitive control enhancement among bilinguals. Future research may include more typical patterns of bilingual language use experience, and wider coverage of the bilingual population including, for example, child bilinguals who grow up with two or more languages in their homes. Another line of further research is to see how distinction of experiences with translation, consecutive, and simultaneous interpreting, may lead to differences in different aspects of cognitive control, which in turn may help explore the exact nature of interpreting training as described in the current experiment and its connection with cognitive control advantages.

6.6 Conclusion

The current experiment has investigated how one of the most important aspects of bilingualism, language interpreting experience, contributes to cognitive control differences among young adult bilinguals when L2 proficiency is manipulated. The results show that L2 proficiency does not contribute significantly to cognitive control differences in inhibition, conflict monitoring or mental set shifting. However, the results also indicate that language interpreting experience, as part of bilinguals' language use ecology, significantly contributes to cognitive control enhancement on the aspect of mental set shifting in young adult bilinguals. Future work may include more examples of specific bilingual experience to further examine the possible relationship between such specific experience and possible enhancement of specific aspects of cognitive control. In next chapter, one more example of specific bilingual experience is to be examined. That is, public speaking experience.

Chapter 7: Experiment Four – Public Speaking Experience and Cognitive Control[15]

7.1 Introduction

Experiment Three has provided evidence showing that bilinguals with interpreting experience have better mental set shifting ability even than control bilinguals who do not have such experience. Therefore, to compare bilinguals differing in language use experiences is very important and may provide a new outlook for examining the nature of bilingual advantage. In the current experiment (**Experiment Four**), we explore another example of bilingual language use experience, i.e., public speaking. If bilingual groups have intensive public speaking experience, rather than language interpreting experience, what will the result be like? This experiment answers *Research Question 4* raised in the current doctoral volume: *Does public speaking experience contribute to cognitive control differences among young adult bilinguals?*

7.2 Specific Background

In Experiment One, it has been shown that bilingualism really does bring about cognitive control advantage in bilinguals, which is consistent with a large body of studies indicating that bilingual experience has a systematic and significant positive impact upon bilinguals' cognitive functioning (Bialystok et al., 2009; Bialystok et al., 2012; Peal & Lambert, 1962). Bilingual experience may "train the brain" and improve performances under conditions of competitive information selection

15 The main content of this experiment has been published in the journal *Bilingualism: Language and Cognition* for publication (2015). doi: 10.1017/S1366728915000474.

(Stocco, Yamasaki, Natalenko, & Prat, 2012), bilingual experience may pose compensatory effects on children's cognitive development, and bilingual experience may differentiate the learning strategy and subsequent neural mechanisms of cognitive control used by bilinguals compared to monolinguals (Bradley et al., 2012; Carlson & Meltzoff, 2008; Kroll & Bialystok, 2013).

However, how a specific bilingual experience leads to change/enhancement of non-verbal cognitive control remains largely unknown. *Experiment Two* has shown that L2 proficiency does not contribute to cognitive control differences in a direct and significant way, although it is possible that greater L2 proficiency gap may bring about the effect. *Experiment Three* has examined the specific role of language interpreting experience in enhancing bilinguals' cognitive control ability, with the manipulation of L2 proficiency. The results show that L2 proficiency does not contribute significantly to cognitive control advantage among bilinguals, but language interpreting experience plays a significant role in enhancing cognitive control among bilinguals. More specifically, this enhancement emerges only in the aspect of mental set shifting but not in conflict monitoring or inhibition, probably because mental set shifting is more closely associated with language interpreting experience. These results provide evidence supporting our *general hypothesis* that *differences in bilingual experiences may lead to different aspects of bilingual advantage in cognitive control*. If this hypothesis is correct, then more comparisons between different bilingual populations, who have different language use experiences, should be done to lend support for such hypothesis. Therefore, characterizing different bilingual experiences will be a crucial step to explore the nature of bilingual advantage.

Unlike language interpreting experience in Experiment Three, public speaking (whether in L1 or L2) for bilinguals is another specific case of bilingual language use experience. On the one hand, when delivering public speech, bilinguals need to select the target language to use and inhibit the interference from the non-target language, and they also need to maintain the goal of speaking the target language as both languages are non-selectively activated. In order to succeed in selecting the target language, bilinguals keep using a language control mechanism (Green, 1998) to deal with competition not only from within-language choices such as semantic neighbors but also from between-language choices such as words for the same concept. In public speaking, bilingual individuals must continuously monitor the context, maintain the task goal, and resist interference from other competing actions that may be triggered by situational context (Green & Abutalebi, 2013). As a result, bilinguals with public speaking experience may become advantageous at some aspects of general cognitive control. Moreover, compared to L1, L2 public speaking (the weaker language) may produce more significant changes/enhancement of cognitive control since in L2 public speaking, speakers need to monitor the appropriate context and exclude interferences from the stronger language, usually their L1.

On the other hand, public speaking is different from speaking in casual context. Particularly, in the public speaking context, bilinguals not only need to monitor the appropriate context for the target language use but also need to inhibit or regulate the performance anxiety from the speech context facing a large audience (Jones, Fazio, & Vasey, 2012). The context of public speaking is an important factor affecting cognitive control. Some studies have suggested a relationship between stress regulation (a form of emotion regulation) and cognitive control in public speaking (e.g., Fineman, 2008). Public speaking evokes fear and anxiety for many people. Some previous studies indicate that in the domain of public speaking, speakers need the ability to self-regulate attentional processes to focus on the current goal and exclude performance anxiety. Inferior performance of public speaking has been reported related to lower attentional control. Attentional control plays as a buffer that helps to reduce performance anxiety (Jones et al., 2012). That is to say, in public speaking, in order to achieve a better performance, speakers are continuously adopting cognitive control to regulate emotion (e.g., fear, stress, or anxiety), such as monitoring the appropriate emotion, inhibiting the irrelevant emotion (Schel & Crone, 2013). If so, the experience of public speaking must contribute to cognitive control enhancement in some significant ways. In previous literature, public speaking (or in adapted forms) has been used as an effective way to induce, assess or treat social anxiety (Bergamaschi et al., 2011; Pribyl, Keaten, & Sakamoto, 2001; Wallach, Safir, & Bar-Zvi, 2009), but few studies have ever directly examined how such experience may affect cognitive control among bilinguals.

Therefore, the purpose of the current experiment is to investigate whether and how public speaking experience may contribute to cognitive control differences among young adults who are homogeneous in L1 and cultural background. Our *hypothesis* for this question is that bilinguals with public speaking experience may significantly contribute to cognitive control differences in some ways, when other factors (such as L2 proficiency) are controlled. In order to find an answer for the question, we speculate that: 1) both L1 and L2 public speaking experience will contribute to cognitive control enhancement, so public speaking bilingual groups may be better than control bilinguals and monolinguals in some aspects of cognitive control. For this purpose, we included the monolingual group and the bilingual group from Experiment One as control groups for comparisons. 2) L2 public speaking bilinguals may perform better than L1 public speaking bilinguals, since L2 public speaking requires a more efficient cognitive control to inhibit the interference from L1, which is a dominant language. For this purpose, we included two bilingual groups who had intensive L1 public speaking training experience or intensive L2 public speaking training experience for comparisons.

Therefore, four groups of participants were included in the current experiment for comparisons with an aim to examine the cognitive control differences among them. There were one monolingual group[16] and three bilingual groups (the L1 public speaking group, the bilingual group[17], the L2 public speaking group). For task consistency, all the participants were required to complete the same three behavioral tasks in the previous experiments of this doctoral research: the Flanker task, the Number Stroop task, and the Wisconsin Card Sorting Test (WCST). The first two tasks, i.e., the Flanker task and the Number Stroop task, aimed to measure the aspects of conflict monitoring and inhibition. Both tasks involve ignoring distracting and conflicting information and inhibiting irrelevant response (Costa et al., 2009; Miyake et al., 2000). The third task, i.e., the WCST, aimed to measure the aspect of mental set shifting.

Our specific predictions for the current experiment are: i) public speaking participants may outperform their counterparts in some or all

16 This group was the same monolingual group from Experiment One.

17 This group was the same bilingual group from Experiment One.

of these tasks; ii) L2 public speaking groups may outperform all the other groups in some or all of these tasks.

7.3 Method

7.3.1 Participants

Three groups of unbalanced young adult Chinese-English bilinguals and one group of monolinguals (42 males/94 females, mean age = 21.27 years, SD = 2.55) participated in this experiment. *The bilingual group* and *the monolingual group* from Experiment One were included here as controls for comparisons. The L1 public speaking group and the L2 public speaking group were the experimental groups in the current experiment. All the bilingual groups were students from a university in China, and *the monolinguals* were junior middle school or high school graduates, who did not receive higher education (as already stated in Experiment One). All the participants were right-handed, reported normal or corrected-to-normal vision and had no speech or hearing disorders. They took part in the experiments either for monetary compensation or for course credits. Participants gave informed consent and their rights were protected in accord with the ethical standards of the university's Academic Board.

The L2 public speaking group and the bilingual group were English major students from the university and had been learning English (as a foreign language) for about 11.87 years. In their university study, they took at least 16 hours of in-class English learning (according to their class schedule) each week for each semester (two semesters in a year). *The L2 public speaking group*, 30 participants altogether, had received extra time of L2 public speaking training for 2.8 years (SD = 0.9), with about 8 hours a week in such training both in and after the training class. They had been trained in two skills: prepared L2 speech and impromptu L2 speech. *The bilingual group* (as stated in Experiment One), 43 participants in all, took normal English major classes but did not receive any formal training in L1/L2 public speaking.

The L1 public speaking group, 30 participants in all, was composed of Chinese Broadcasting major students. They received L1 public speaking training for a mean time of 2.9 years (SD=0.3). Their training tasks included news broadcasting, prepared speech, impromptu speech, and simulated TV show hosting, taking about 9 hours each week according to their class schedule. Their English study time was limited to around 3 hours of in-class learning each week (few reported extra learning after class because they were not required to do so).

All the groups were required to complete a composite questionnaire concerning participants' L2 learning background and L2 proficiency[18]. L2 proficiency, composed of listening, speaking, reading, and writing, was self-rated on a 10-point Likert scale (same as the one in Experiment 1), which is a widely recognized measurement in bilingual research and is significantly correlated with objective measurements of language proficiency (Marian et al., 2007; Prior & Gollan, 2011). As objective measurement of L2 proficiency, English (L2) verbal fluency test (as in Experiment 1) was adopted, in which all participants were required to produce as many words as possible within one minute according to the categories presented (jobs, sports, animals). Category fluency has been reported to be strongly indicative of vocabulary size (Bialystok et al., 2009). For objective test of Intelligence, all participants took Ravens Advanced Progressive Matrices (as in Experiment 1) (Raven et al., 1977), which consists of 72 items grouped in six types. In each type there are 12 items. Each item is composed of a pattern with a missing part in the lower right. Participants were required to select the right one from a set of six or eight alternatives to complete the pattern within 40 minutes. Correct answers were counted as intelligence scores. Table 14 has summarized the main characteristics of all these participants' background information[19].

---

18 Participants' L1, as native language, was considered homogeneously highly proficient as they were from a similar linguistic and cultural background, but we admit that there might be subtle variations.

19 All the participants came from similar family and cultural background, so we assumed they had similar socioeconomic status (SES) although there might be variations. Furthermore, Hook et al. (2013) suggested an association between SES and cognitive control, this association is mostly based on child bilinguals (but see Prior & Gollan, 2011).

Table 14. Participant characteristics in language history, language proficiency, and language experience etc. across public speaking and control groups.

	Monolingual *n=33*	*L1 Speaking* *n=30*	*L2 Speaking* *n=30*	*Bilingual* *n=43*
Age	21.5 ^{b} (3.6)	19.5^{a} (1.0)	21.2 ^{b}(2.3)	22.4 ^{c} (1.8)
Education (years)	11.3 ^{a} (2.4)	13.5^{b} (1.0)	15.2 ^{c} (2.3)	16.4 ^{d} (1.8)
Raven's Matrices	65.2 (5.5)	65.4 (4.9)	65.0 (5.0)	64.7 (4.1)
L2 Learning History (years)	4.1 ^{a} (1.2)	11.8 ^{b} (1.7)	11.2 ^{b} (2.3)	12.4 ^{c} (1.7)
L2/L1 speaking Training (years)	0.0	2.9 (0.3)	2.8 (0.9)	0.0
L2 Proficiency	7.1 ^{a}(2.9)	19.5 ^{b} (4.4)	24.5^{c}(4.3)	23.2^{c}(4.5)
L2 Verbal Category Fluency	6.7 ^{a} (1.7)	19.1 ^{b} (8.1)	25.2^{c}(5.2)	24.4^{c}(4.2)
L2 Exposure (%)	0.0	7.6^{a} (3.4)	41.1 ^{b}(20.8)	43.3^{b} (17.7)
L2 Speaking (%)	0.0	8.8^{a} (9.1)	27.2^{c} (13.4)	16.9 ^{b}(10.3)

Note: Means in the same row with different superscript letters differ from each other significantly at p<.01 or .05. The total percentage of L1 and L2 equals 100; the total score for L2 proficiency is 40; the total score for L2 using frequency is 60.

First, *the L2 public speaking group* and *the bilingual group*, matched on self-rated L2 proficiency, English verbal (category) fluency, and L2 exposure, differed in the history of L2 learning (11.2 *vs.* 12.4) (p=.011) and L2 speaking (27.2 vs. 16.9) (p<.001)[20]. Second, *the L2 public speaking group* and *the bilingual group* had a higher L2 proficiency, higher L2 exposure, and higher L2 speaking than *the L1 public speaking group* and *the monolingual group* (ps<.001). Third, all the groups did not differ in intelligence measures (Raven's Matrices) although there were differences on education years across groups. Finally, the groups differed in age statistically, but it's not practically significant or relevant to our concern because all the groups were between 21–23 years, a period which is at the peak of cognitive functioning for all the participants.

20 As reported by the participants, *the L2 public speaking group* spoke L2 for more time mainly because they had extra hours of L2 public speaking training.

7.3.2 Materials and Procedures

The experiment lasted for approximately 1.5 hours. Participants completed two sets of test. The first set was a composite questionnaire (as stated above), and the second was three computerized cognitive control tasks: the Flanker task, the Number Stroop task, and the Wisconsin Card Sorting Test (WCST).

Cognitive Control Tasks
The tasks (the Flanker task, the Number Stroop task, and the WCST task) were the same ones adopted in previous experiments of the current doctoral research (as in Experiment One, Experiment Two, and Experiment Three).

7.4 Result

7.4.1 Data Trimming

In the tasks of Flanker and Number Stroop, data of erroneous and extreme responses were first excluded, and then trials that fell above 3 standard deviations (SDs) of the overall mean for each subject (in each condition) in all the three tasks were then eliminated, accounting for 2.17% of the total correct responses. In the WCST task, additional variables such as completed categories, overall errors and types of errors were analyzed respectively to investigate group differences.

7.4.2 Flanker Task

Table 15 presents the data for the Flanker task performance across groups. Three participants from the groups were excluded because of false operations in the task. Two indices were used to compare between-group performances. The first one is Flanker conflict, the difference in mean response times between trials that require conflict resolution (incongruent) compared to those that do not (congruent). Smaller Flanker conflict implies superior ability in conflict resolution, thus stronger ability of inhibition (Bialystok et al., 2004; Bialystok et al., 2008; Costa et al., 2009; Paap & Greenberg, 2013). The second one is overall RTs in each condition, which reflects global goal-oriented maintenance and conflict monitoring. Faster RTs means superior performance in conflict monitoring. Bilingual advantage in overall RTs may reveal bilinguals' better ability to handle tasks that involve mixing trials of different types, i.e. the efficiency of monitoring system (Costa et al., 2009; Costa et al., 2008; Martin-Rhee & Bialystok, 2008).

Table 15. Means (standard deviations) of reaction times in Flanker conditions and means of Flanker conflict across public speaking and control groups.

	Monolingual *n=32*	*L1 Speaking* *n=30*	*L2 Speaking* *n=28*	*Bilingual* *n=43*
Flanker Neutral	549.3[b] (90.8)	481.3[a](71.9)	479.5[a] (47.5)	536.0[b](91.3)
Flanker Incongruent	589.7[b] (88.3)	525.6[a](78.4)	523.3[a] (56.4)	578.3[b](87.1)
Flanker Congruent	530.3[b](106.4)	465.4[a](78.3)	464.5[a] (55.5)	516.4[b] (80.6)
Flanker Conflict*	59.4 (39.7)	60.2 (34.0)	58.8 (23.6)	61.9 (49.5)

Note: Means in the same row with different superscript letters differ from each other significantly at p<.01 or .05. *Flanker conflict means the different response times between incongruent condition and congruent condition.

We conducted a repeated measures analysis of variance (ANOVA) with Group (the monolingual group, the L1 public speaking group, the bilingual group, and the L2 public speaking group) as between-subject variable and condition (neutral, incongruent, congruent) as within-subject variable. This analysis revealed a significant main effect of condition, F (2, 258) =178.344, p<.001, η^2=.580, but there was no condition and group interaction (F<1). Planned comparisons showed that participants responded more quickly on the neutral condition (514.97ms) than on the incongruent condition (557.56), F (1,129) =177.800, p<.001. Participants responded more quickly on the congruent condition (497.30) than on the neutral condition (514.97), F (1, 129) =30.523, p<.001, and than on the incongruent condition (557.56), F (1,129) =301.008, p<.001, reflecting significant Flanker effect. Importantly, the main effect of group was significant, F (3, 129) =6.453, p<.001, η^2=.130, with the L1 and L2 public speaking groups performing faster than the monolingual group and the bilingual group in the three conditions of the Flanker task.

ANOVA analysis results showed that there were no group differences on the Flanker conflict ($F<1$), but there were group differences of global RTs in all the three conditions: congruent F (3,129) =5.404, p=.002; neutral F (3,129) =6.639, p<.001; incongruent F (3,129) =6.009, p=.001. Post-hoc analysis showed that L2 public speaking group was faster than the bilingual group and the monolingual group in neutral condition (p=.004, p=.001 respectively), incongruent condition (p=.005, p=.002 respectively), and congruent condition (p=.011, p=.003 respectively). L1 public speaking group was faster than the bilingual group and the monolingual group in neutral condition (p=.005, p=.001 respectively), incongruent condition (p=.006, p=.002 respectively), and congruent condition (p=.011, p=.002 respectively). Nevertheless, there were no group differences between L1 and L2 speaking groups (ps>.910), and no group differences between the monolingual group and the bilingual group (ps>.470).

To be more cautious, in order to further confirm the role of public speaking experience in enhancing cognitive control, we conducted further analyses. We entered public speaking experience (two continuous levels: 1=public speaking; 0=non-speaking), L2 proficiency, L2 history, years of education, L2 exposure, and L2 speaking as independent variables to conduct regression analyses in the three conditions of the Flanker task. The multiple regression models were significant for the congruent condition (adjusted R^2=.093, F (6, 120) =3.149, p=.007), the neutral condition (adjusted R^2=.099, F (6, 120) =3.299, p=.005), and the incongruent condition (adjusted R^2=.107, F (6, 120) =3.525, p=.003). More specifically, the results showed that L2 proficiency, L2 history, years of education, L2 exposure, and L2 speaking did not contribute significantly to the effects (congruent condition: p=.671, p=.519,

p=.216, p=.642, p=.605 respectively; neutral condition: p=.918, p=.793, p=.420, p=.803, p=.461 respectively; incongruent condition: p=.523, p=.997, p=.322, p=.921, p=.266 respectively), whereas public speaking experience contribute significantly to the effects in all conditions (congruent condition: p=.005; neutral condition: p=.004; incongruent condition: p=.004).

To sum up, as is already shown in Experiment One, the control bilingual group, who did not have public speaking experience, does not outperform the control monolingual group. Moreover, the two public speaking groups, matched on public speaking experience but differing in L2 proficiency, perform similarly in the flanker task. However, the fact that both the L1 and L2 public speaking groups outperform the monolingual and the bilingual groups in the global RTs in each condition indicates that public speaking experience (whether in L1 or in L2) significantly contributes to conflict monitoring. The results of multiple regression analyses further confirm this finding.

7.4.3 Number Stroop Task

Two participants from the monolingual group, four from the L1 public speaking group, five from the L2 public speaking group, and two from the bilingual group were excluded because of false operations. Table 16 lists the detailed descriptive data of these group performances in the Number Stroop task.

Like what we did in analyzing the Flanker task performance, similar indices (global RTs and Stroop conflict) were compared in order to examine the performance differences across these groups. A repeated measures analysis of variance was conducted, with group (the monolingual group, the L1 public speaking group, the bilingual group, the L2 pubic speaking group) as between-subject variables and condition (neutral, incongruent, congruent) as within-subject variables.

Table 16. Means (standard deviations) of reaction times in the Number Stroop conditions, and means (standard deviations) of Number Stroop conflict across public speaking and control groups.

	Monolingual *n=31*	*L1 Speaking* *n=26*	*L2 Speaking* *n=25*	*Bilingual* *n=41*
Number Stroop Neutral	721.8[b] (119.3)	721.21[b] (85.0)	663.6[a] (59.2)	735.9[b](107.9)
Number Stroop Incongruent	712.5 (95.2)	735.6[b] (111.2)	674.2[a] (82.2)	732.7[b] (98.3)
Number Stroop Congruent	693.2[b*] (100.0)	689. 7[b]*(79.6)	646.3[a] (86.0)	693.7[b](95.9)
Number Stroop Conflict*	19.3 (50.7)	45.9(68.1)	27.9 (45.0)	39.0 (64.3)

Note: Means in the same row with different superscript letters differ from each other significantly at $p<.01$ or .05, but b* means the significance is at a marginal level or having a tendency ($p<.10$). Number Stroop conflict* means the different response times between incongruent condition and congruent condition.

This analysis revealed a significant main effect of condition, F (2, 238) =22.828, $p<.001$, $\eta^2=.161$, but there was no condition and group interaction, F (6, 238) =1.064, $p=.385$. The results of planned comparisons showed that participants responded more quickly on congruent condition (683.10ms) than on neutral condition (714.53ms), F (1, 119)=33.852, $p<.001$, and on incongruent condition (716.32ms), F (1, 119) = 37.787, $p<.001$, reflecting significant Stroop effect. But participants did not respond more quickly on neutral condition (714.53ms) than on incongruent condition (716.32ms), F(1,119)=.304, $p=.582$. Test of between-subject effects in all three conditions together showed that the main effect of participant group was marginally significant, F (3, 119) =2.525, $p=.061$, $\eta^2=.051$, suggesting that there might be differences across these groups in the Number Stroop task. Post-hoc analysis of ANOVA showed that in congruent condition, L2 public speaking performed with a faster tendency than L1 public speaking group ($p=.094$), faster than the bilingual group ($p=.044$), and faster than the monolingual group (marginal $p=.060$). However, there were no differences across all the other groups (the L1 public speaking group vs. the bilingual group, $p=.862$; the L1 public speaking group vs. the monolingual group, $p=.887$; the bilingual group vs. the monolingual group, p=.980). In neutral condition, L2 public speaking performed faster than the L1 public speaking group (p=.039), the bilingual group (p=.005), and the monolingual group (p=.030). Meanwhile, there were no differences across all the other groups (the L1 public speaking group vs. the bilingual group, p=.554; the L1 public speaking group vs. the monolingual group, p=.983; the bilingual group vs. the monolingual group, p=.549). In incongruent condition, the L2 public speaking group performed faster than the L1 public speaking group (p=.026), and the bilingual group (p=.020), but not the monolingual group (p=.146). At the same time, there were no differences across all the other groups (the L1 public speaking group vs. the bilingual group, p=.906; the L1 public speaking group vs. the monolingual group, p=.375; the bilingual group vs. the monolingual group, p=.386). The ANOVA analysis of Number Stroop conflict showed that there were no group differences across the four groups (F (3,119) =1.182, p=.320).

Similarly, in order to further clarify the role of public speaking experience in cognitive control differences, we conducted multiple regression analyses by entering public speaking experience (two continuous levels: 1=public speaking; 0=non-speaking), L2 proficiency, L2 history, years of education, L2 exposure, and L2 speaking as independent variables to examine the effects in the three conditions of the Flanker task. The multiple regression models were significant (or marginally significant) for the congruent condition (adjusted R^2=.040, F (6, 114) =2.248, p=.068), for the neutral condition (adjusted R^2=.077, F (6, 114) =3.520, p=.009), but not for the incongruent condition (adjusted R^2=.027, F (6, 114) =1.840, p=.126). More specifically, the results showed that L2 proficiency, L2 history, years of education, L2 exposure, and L2 speaking did not contribute significantly to the effects (congruent condition: p=.542, p=.127, p=.163, p=.884, p=.533 respectively; neutral condition: p=.587, p=.105, p=.181, p=.879, p=.758 respectively; incongruent condition: p=.957, p=.155, p=.168, p=.853, p=.482 respectively), whereas public speaking experience contribute significantly to the effects in each condition (congruent condition: p=.023; neutral condition: p=.001; incongruent condition: p=.024). These results are consistent with the ANOVA analyses.

The results are consistent with our predictions. L2 public speaking group perform significantly faster than the other three groups (L1 public speaking group, the bilingual group, and the monolingual group) in the Number Stroop task on one or more conditions in terms of global RTs, but not in conflict resolution. However, there are no group differences across L1 public speaking group, the bilingual group, and the monolingual group. Along with previous results, the fact that L2 public speaking group outperform L1 public speaking group (matched on the public speaking experience) leads us to conclude that public speaking experience, particularly L2 public speaking, significantly contributes to conflict monitoring in cognitive control.

7.4.4 WCST

Unlike the Flanker task and the Number Stroop task (which measured inhibitory control and conflict monitoring in cognitive control), the WCST task was used to detect the ability of mental set shifting (mental flexibility) in cognitive control. In this test, we report analyses on global performance (global RTs, number of completed categories and overall errors) and different types of errors (perseverative errors, previous category errors) to capture the performance differences in mental flexibility (Barceló & Knight, 2002; Yudes et al., 2011). Table 17 presents the means and standard deviations of the global RTs, the number of completed categories, overall errors, perseverative errors, and previous category errors across groups.

Global performance. We conducted ANOVA to compare group differences in performing the task of WCST. The ANOVA analysis of global RTs showed that there were no differences across the groups, F (3,131) =1.510, p=.215, reflecting that all the groups responded with similar speed to sort the implied rule in the WCST task (see Table 17).

Table 17. Means (standard deviations) of global performance and types of errors in the WCST across public speaking and control groups.

	Monolingual *n=32*	*L1 Speaking* *n=30*	*L2 Speaking* *n=30*	*Bilingual* *n=43*
Global RTs	1383.7(549.8)	1354.9(450.9)	1347.4(429.7)	1555.5(526.3)
Completed Categories	5.7^{a} (2.8)	6.4^{a}(3.2)	8.8^{b} (3.3)	9.2^{b} (3.4)
Overall errors	73.2^{b}(13.4)	70.3^{b}(15.1)	58.2^{a} (14.3)	57.7^{a} (14.1)
Perseverative errors	54.4^{b}(15.4)	50.0^{b}(16.9)	37.7^{a} (16.1)	37.3^{a} (15.3)
Previous Category errors	41.6^{c}(17.7)	30.5^{b}(18.0)	20.3^{a} (15.7)	19.9^{a} (13.1)

Note: Means in the same row with different superscript letters differ from each other significantly at p<.01 or .05.

The second indicator of WCST performance was how many correct categories the participants completed. In this WCST task, the number of categories ranged from 0 to 19. "0" means that the participant was not able to complete at least 5 consecutive correct responses to trials of any category, and "19" means that the participant successfully completed trials of all the categories. The results of ANOVA analysis on the number of completed categories indicated that there were significant group differences across the groups, F (3, 131) =10.155, p<.001, η^2=.189. The results of multiple comparisons showed that both the L2 public speaking group and the bilingual group completed a higher number of completed categories than the L1 public speaking group (p=.004, p<.001 respectively) and the monolingual group (ps<.001). However, there was no group difference between the L2 public speaking group and the bilingual (p=.656), and no group difference between the L1 public speaking group and the monolingual group (p=.364).

As for the number of overall errors committed in executing WCST, the results of ANOVA showed that there were significant group differences across the groups, F (3, 131)=10.769, p<.001, η^2=.199. Post-hoc tests showed that the L2 public speaking group and the bilingual group committed fewer errors than the L1 public speaking group (p=.001, p<.001 respectively) and the monolingual group (ps<.001). However, there was no group difference between the L2 public speaking group and the bilingual group (p=.882), and no group difference between the L1 public speaking group and the monolingual group (p=.428).

Types of errors. When assessing WCST performance, we usually distinguish between perseverative errors and non-perseverative errors (Heaton et al., 1993). Perseverative errors are failures to change the mental rule after receiving negative feedback so that the person continues sorting the cards according to the previous-category dimension despite feedback indicating that the response was wrong (Yudes et al., 2011). And perseverative errors can be further categorized into perseverations to the immediately preceding category and perseverations to a different-category (Hartman et al., 2001; Hartman et al., 2003; Yudes et al., 2011). Previous category perseverations reflect lack of flexibility to change the mental set to a new rule, while different category perseverations reflect the understanding that the previous rule is no longer correct but there is an unsuccessful attempt to infer a new rule.

The results of ANOVAs showed there were significant differences across the groups on the number of perseverative errors, F (3, 131) =9.990, p<.001, η^2=.187. Post-hoc tests showed that the L2 public speaking group and the bilingual group committed fewer perseverative errors than the L1 public speaking group (p=.003, p=.001 respectively) and the monolingual group (ps<.001). However, there was no group difference between the L2 public speaking group and the bilingual group (p=.907), and no group difference between L1 public speaking group and the monolingual group (p=.286).

On pervious category errors, an ANOVA test showed that there were significant differences across the groups, F (3, 131) =13.111, p<.001, η^2=.235. The results of pairwise comparisons showed that the L2 public speaking group and the bilingual group committed fewer previous category errors than the L1 public speaking group (p=.015, p=.006 respectively) and the monolingual group (ps<.001). However, there was no group difference between the L2 public speaking group and the bilingual group (p=.922), but L1 public speaking group had fewer such errors than the monolingual group (p=.009).

Further analysis. To sum up, there are three major findings in the above analysis. First, the L2 public speaking group and the bilingual group, matched on L2 proficiency and L2 exposure but differing in L2 speaking (mainly as a result of L2 public speaking training), are not different from each other in the performance of WCST. Second, between the two public speaking groups that were matched on public speaking training but differed in L2 proficiency, the L2 public speaking group with higher L2 proficiency outperform the L1 public speaking group with lower L2 proficiency in the WCST task. Third, all the bilingual groups (the L2 public speaking group, the bilingual group, the L1 pubic speaking group) outperform the monolingual group in the WCST task. Taken together, the three findings suggest that it is L2 proficiency instead of public speaking training that has significantly contributed to mental set shifting enhancement in cognitive control.

And yet, to be more cautious, in order to further clarify the role of L2 proficiency in the WCST performance, we conducted multiple regression analyses by entering L2 proficiency, public speaking experience (classified into two levels: one with public speaking "1" and the other without "0"), L2 history, years of education, L2 exposure, and L2 speaking as independent variables and WCST performances as dependent variables. The results showed that the multiple regression models were significant for "completed categories" (adjusted R^2=.181, F (6,122) =5.718, p<.001), "overall errors" (adjusted R^2=.154, F (6,122)=4.847, p<.001), "perseverative errors" (adjusted R^2=.126, F (6,122)=4.053, p=.001), and "previous category errors" (adjusted R^2=.187, F (6,122)=5.792, p<.001). More specifically, public speaking experience, L2 history, years of education, L2 exposure, and L2 speaking did not significantly contribute to the differences ("completed categories", p=.361, p=.298, p=.199, p=.494, p=.347 respectively; "overall errors", p=.452, p=.285, p=.205, p=.575, p=.522 respectively; "perseverative errors", p=.535, p=.459, p=.247, p=.678, p=.734 respectively; "previous category errors", p=.351, p=.541, p=.955, p=.976, p=960 respectively). However, L2 proficiency significantly contributed to the group differences on all the indexes ("completed categories", p=.003; "overall errors", p=.006; "perseverative errors", p=.022; "previous category errors", p=.012). All these results are consistent with previous ANOVA analyses and indicate that bilingualism (or L2 proficiency), rather than public speaking (or other factors), have made major contributions to cognitive control enhancement in mental set shifting.

7.5 Discussion

The purpose of the current experiment is to examine the contribution of public speaking experience to cognitive control differences among young adult bilinguals/monolinguals. Previous studies suggest that bilinguals have advantages over monolinguals in cognitive control (Barac & Bialystok, 2012; Bialystok et al., 2009; Bialystok et al., 2012; Gold et al., 2013), due to the fact that bilinguals have the experience of continuously using language control mechanism to monitor language processing such as inhibiting non-target language and switching between two languages (Barac & Bialystok, 2012; Bradley et al., 2012; Green, 2011; Stocco et al., 2012). In public speaking, bilinguals need to monitor the appropriate context, maintain the goal and inhibit the unwanted non-target language. Moreover, public speaking requires the bilingual speakers to inhibit the unwanted emotions such as anxiety in delivering a public speech (Jones et al., 2012). Therefore, the long term practice of public speaking may greatly reduce anxiety (Bergamaschi et al., 2011; Pribyl et al., 2001) and thus also lead to cognitive control advantage. The current experiment compares cognitive control differences among four different bilingual and monolingual groups (L1 public speaking group, L2 public speaking group, bilingual group, and monolingual group) by administering three tasks (the Flanker task, the Number Stroop task, and the WCST task) that measure different aspects of cognitive control: inhibition, conflict monitoring and mental set shifting. We hypothesize that public speaking experience may lead to specific aspect of enhancement in cognitive control, compared with control groups.

The experimental results support our hypothesis. The main results of ANOVA and regression analyses are summarized in the following paragraphs:

i. The result that the L1 public speaking group and the L2 public speaking group outperform the bilingual group and the monolingual group in the Flanker task in terms of global RTs, and the result that the L2 public speaking group outperform the bilingual group, the monolingual group and the L1 public speaking group in the Number Stroop task in terms of global RTs collaboratively show that public speaking experience significantly contributes to the enhancement of *conflict monitoring* in cognitive control, with L2 public speaking playing a more powerful role in such enhancement.

ii) In the WCST task that tests *mental set shifting*, all the bilingual groups (the L2 public speaking group, the bilingual group, and the L1 public speaking group) outperform the monolingual group in one or more indicators. Moreover, the group with higher L2 proficiency perform significantly better than the group with lower L2 proficiency (both L2 proficiency and performance: *L2 public speaking=bilingual>L1 public speaking>monolingual*). This result is also consistent with the regression analysis, which shows that L2 proficiency significantly predicts the WCST performance. These results altogether suggest that L2 proficiency, rather than public speaking experience, mainly contributes to mental set shifting differences in cognitive control.

Importantly, these results indicate that bilingual advantage is closely associated with the specific features of language use experiences and that only certain specific aspect(s) of cognitive control related to language use experience can be significantly affected. Our experiments results show that L2 proficiency contributes most to mental set shifting whereas public speaking contributes most to conflict monitoring in cognitive control. Furthermore, L2 public speaking contributes more significantly than L1 public speaking to conflict monitoring in cognitive control. These results are consistent with the lately proposed hypothesis that "language control processes themselves adapt to the recurrent demands placed on them by the interactional context" (the adaptive control hypothesis) (Green & Abutalebi, 2013). Similar ideas have also been discussed by other researchers (Kroll & Bialystok, 2013; Luk & Bialystok, 2013) that the diversity of bilingual experience modulates the effect of bilingual advantage.

As reasoned in the rationale, for bilinguals, the experience of intensive training in public speaking, which requires speakers to monitor and focus attentively only on the target language and/or to inhibit interference from the other language and speaking anxiety, may significantly affect cognitive control. According to the results of the Flanker task and the Number Stroop task, this particular experience greatly enhances bilinguals' ability of conflict monitoring in cognitive control. In the context of public speaking, bilinguals must be aware that they need to deliver a speech only in the target language. Therefore, the first step they need to do is to monitor the appropriate use of the target language, or to maintain the goal. If the target language is L2, the demand of monitoring should be higher because L1 poses a stronger interference. This explains the more significant effect of L2 public speaking experience in conflict monitoring in the current experiment. The other source of conflict monitoring enhancement may result from the need to monitor and regulate emotion (reduce anxiety) in public speaking, in which individuals experience anxious thoughts, dysfunctional beliefs, and excessive fears of negative evaluation (Harb, Eng, Zaider, & Heimberg, 2003). Recent neurocognitive data show that in emotion regulation and cognitive control, there is the common involvement of ACC that plays a crucial role in both emotion and cognitive control and in the interactions between them (Mueller, 2011). All of these consistently explain why intensive practice of public speaking experience can strengthen speakers' cognitive control in the current experiment.

However, why didn't the public speaking groups outperform the control groups in the Flanker conflict or the Number Stroop conflict (inhibition)? A smaller conflict indicates a better ability of conflict resolution. Very likely, the reason lies in the specific and unique language use context of public speaking. Once the goal maintenance (speaking one language) has been achieved, the interfering information (the other language) is kept at a relatively stable but low activation level, thus offering no need of efficient conflict resolution. Previous studies suggest that bilinguals outperform monolinguals in inhibitory control (inhibition) only when the task requires the participants to adjust continuously to the different demands associated to different types of trials (Costa et al., 2009). Obviously, keeping one goal (speaking one language) without continuously changing to different demands (changing to the other language) requires monitoring and maintaining the goal but not resolving conflict.

The results of WCST can also be justified. Firstly, the two high L2 proficiency matched bilingual groups (the L2 pubic speaking group and the bilingual group) outperform the two low L2 proficiency groups (the L1 public speaking group and the monolingual group), which consistently confirms the role of L2 proficiency in mental set shifting (Bialystok & Martin, 2004; Bialystok & Viswanathan, 2009; Marzecová et al., 2013; Yudes et al., 2011). This result seems contradictory to the results in Experiments 2 and 3, but it is consistent to our speculation that greater magnitude of differences in L2 proficiency is more likely to bring about differences in cognitive control (more discussions concerning L2 proficiency will be elaborated in next chapter). Additionally, it is reasonable to state that bilinguals have a more intensive and practical need to switch between different language mental sets whereas monolinguals do not. Similarly, higher L2 proficiency bilinguals may switch more often than lower L2 proficiency bilinguals. Secondly, the fact that the L2 public speaking group and the bilingual group (matched on L2 proficiency) did not differ in the WCST performance shows that public speaking experience does not significantly contribute to mental set shifting. This may be explained by the fact that neither group has intensive training experience of language switching (switching back and forth between the two alternate languages intentionally in practice or communication as the interpreting bilinguals in Experiment Three), which requires efficient involvement of mental set shifting in cognitive control (The L2 public speaking group, as mentioned above, did not need to frequently switch between two languages). Probably, the lack of such experience in language switching for both groups leads to similar performances in the WCST task. Taken together, all these results suggest that bilinguals (and monolinguals) have cognitive control differences only in some specific aspect(s) due to bilinguals' specific experience of language use.

The results in the current experiment (Experiment Four) provide implications for the hot topic of bilingual advantage in cognitive control. Firstly, the current experiment is an attempt to sort out some specific source of bilingualism that may cause cognitive control enhancement in bilinguals. There have been many studies showing that bilinguals gain relative advantage compared to monolinguals in cognitive control. However, it is still unknown what about bilingualism serves as a fundamental source of bilingual advantage. Comparing different groups of bilingual populations with differing language use experiences (Prior & Gollan, 2011) is helpful to find out specific origins of bilingual advantage in cognitive control. Secondly, the incoherence in previous studies (Paap & Greenberg, 2013) may be caused by the heterogeneity of bilingual language use experiences in different bilingual contexts and by the complexity of cognitive control measurement. Many studies did not replicate Bialystok's findings that bilinguals outperform monolinguals in cognitive control, particularly among young bilinguals who are at the peak of their cognition in behavior research. The reason may lie in the fact that language use experience was not adequately taken into consideration. However, by taking specific language use experience as one crucial factor, the current experiment has explored the relationship between specific elements of bilingualism and specific aspects of cognitive control and found that only specific aspect of cognitive control is influenced under the context of a certain specific bilingual language use experience in bilingualism. Although there are many papers formulating the nature of bilingual advantages (e.g., Dong & Li, 2014), comparing different groups of bilingual populations with differing language use experiences (Prior & Gollan, 2011) as we have done in the current research may help find out more. Therefore, future studies are encouraged to specify the exact aspect of cognitive control related to specific bilingual language use experience.

7.6 Conclusion

We conclude that bilingualism indeed contributes to cognitive control enhancement, but in varied ways. Higher L2 proficiency (of bilingualism) is associated with better mental set shifting. However, public speaking experience, whether in L1 or L2, contributes greatly to conflict monitoring in cognitive control, and L2 public speaking has a greater contribution probably because general bilingualism and public speaking experience work together to affect cognitive control. Therefore, different bilingual experiences contribute significantly to cognitive control, but in different aspects. These results suggest a strong relationship between bilinguals' specific language experience and cognitive control advantages. Further follow-up studies are encouraged to identify the specificity of bilingual language experience and its possible effect on specific aspect(s) of cognitive control (Paap, 2014).

Chapter 8: General Discussion

In order to examine the current findings with reference to the literature, this chapter firstly concludes and discusses the experiments results. Secondly the chapter elaborates how specific bilingual experience may be related to specific aspects of bilingual advantage in cognitive control. Finally the chapter highlights the issues related to the incoherence problem of bilingual advantage.

8.1 Summary of the Results

The purpose of the experiments designed in this volume is to further investigate the issue of bilingual advantage by using a new perspective – examining the relationship between specific aspects of bilingual experience in ecology (language use ecology) and specific aspects of cognitive control. This volume hypothesizes that bilingual advantage is closely related to the way in which bilingual languages are used in a specific language context.

The four experiments included in this volume provide new evidence in response to several questions regarding cognitive control advantage as related to bilingualism. In all, these experiments results in the current research provide evidence supporting the existence of bilingual advantage, but, more importantly, these results demonstrate that different bilingual experiences influence different aspects of bilingual advantage in cognitive control (see Table 18).

In ***Experiment One***, in order to verify the existence of bilingual advantage, one young-adult bilingual group and one young-adult monolingual group are compared. In the three tasks measuring conflict monitoring, inhibition, and mental set shifting, the bilinguals do not differ from the monolinguals in the Flanker task and the Number Stroop task, which measure conflict monitoring and inhibition, but the bilinguals do show significant advantage relative to the monolinguals in the WCST task, which measures mental set shifting. These results provide novel evidence of bilingual advantage among young-adult unbalanced Chinese-English bilinguals, who are homogeneous with the monolinguals in demographic, linguistic and cultural backgrounds. Moreover, these results show that the bilingual group was not superior to the monolingual group in the aspects of conflict monitoring and inhibition. It is reasonable to assume that this is because the bilingual group did not have sufficient relevant bilingual experiences prerequisite for advantages in conflict monitoring or inhibition.

The results of ***Experiment One*** in this volume are consistent with previous findings that bilinguals have advantage over monolinguals in cognitive control (Barac, Bialystok, Castro, & Sanchez, 2014; Bialystok et al., 2009; Kroll & Bialystok, 2013). This experiment is new in at least two ways. First, it investigates bilingual advantage using a homogeneous sample of bilinguals, who are young-adult unbalanced Chinese-English participants. In most previous studies, the bilingual subjects were primarily immigrants living in an English-dominant society, and the immigrant status and native/second language were not controlled (e.g., Bialystok et al., 2008; Paap & Greenberg, 2013). Second, it investigates bilingual advantage using a number of tasks that measure separate aspects of cognitive control, whereas most of the previous studies measured only one aspect by using only one single task (Bialystok et al., 2005; Bialystok et al., 2004; Bialystok et al., 2006; Bialystok et al., 2005; Kousaie & Phillips, 2012a). These results provide further evidence of the existence of bilingual advantage and suggest that bilingual advantage may be present universally but only in specific aspect(s) of cognitive control under certain circumstances.

In ***Experiment Two***, in order to examine whether different bilingual experiences contribute to different aspects of bilingual advantage, two young-adult bilingual groups differing in L2 proficiency are compared by administering the same three tasks as adopted in Experiment One; the Flanker task, the Number Stroop task, and the WCST task. Inconsistent with our expectation, each of the three tasks produced a null effect. The bilingual group with higher L2 proficiency did not perform better than the bilingual group with lower L2 proficiency in these tasks.

The results of ***Experiment Two*** are not consistent with some studies in previous research which show that L2 proficiency greatly influences cognitive control in bilinguals (Iluz-Cohen & Armon-Lotem, 2013; Mishra et al., 2012; Singh & Mishra, 2012; Videsott et al., 2012). However, this result raises two important issues. First, language proficiency (usually L2) does not show to what extent bilingualism shall be enough for bilingual advantage to emerge in cognitive control. Second, language use, along with language proficiency, may contribute collaboratively or interactively to cognitive control differences, as bilinguals use their languages in different ways.

With the factor of specific bilingual language use experiences taken into consideration, *Experiment Three* and *Experiment Four* present a clearer picture of what aspects of cognitive control may be enhanced as a result of specific bilingual language-use experience.

In ***Experiment Three***, with L2 proficiency manipulated, the bilingual groups who differed in language interpreting experience were compared with control groups by using the same cognitive control tasks as used in previous studies (the Flanker, the Number Stroop, and the WCST). The results show that L2 proficiency does not contribute significantly to cognitive control differences in all tasks, whereas language interpreting experience contributes significantly to cognitive control differences in the WCST. Bilingual groups with language interpreting experience perform far better than control bilingual groups in the WCST which tests mental set shifting, but not in the Flanker and the Number Stroop tasks which test conflict monitoring and inhibition.

Although the results of ***Experiment Three*** show the limited role of L2 proficiency in affecting cognitive control in the three aspects measured by the Flanker task, the Number Stroop task, and the WCST task, the results are consistent with several recent studies revealing that interpreters demonstrate higher ability in cognitive control in the aspect of mental set shifting but not inhibition (Yudes et al., 2011). By using fMRI, it is indicated that there is similarity between the network underlying bilingual language control and general cognitive control and interpreting experience may strengthen the day-to-day demands of language control so the neural correlates of the brain activity which are shared by general cognitive control are enhanced (Hervais-Adelman et al., 2014). Similar to the results of ***Experiment Three***, another recent study shows that interpreters outperform a control group even in the aspect of updating through the N-back task, but not in the aspect of conflict resolution (inhibition) through the ANTI-V task (Morales, Padilla, et al., 2015). Taken together, all these results suggest that cognitive control enhancement among bilinguals is closely related to specific bilingual language-use experiences, and only experience-dependent aspects of cognitive control are enhanced.

In **Experiment Four**, the public speaking groups and the control groups were compared by using the same three cognitive control tasks adopted in previous experiments of this research. The results demonstrate that the bilinguals with public speaking experience, particularly L2 public speaking experience, are superior to the control bilinguals and monolinguals in the aspect of conflict monitoring measured by the Flanker task and the Number Stroop task. Moreover, unlike the results from Experiments Two and Three, the bilinguals with higher L2 proficiency are better in mental set shifting (measured by the WCST) than the bilinguals with lower L2 proficiency or the monolinguals.

The results of ***Experiment Four*** are consistent with the view that cognitive control enhancement is related to the behavioral ecology of bilingual language use (Green, 2011). How languages are used may distinctively affect cognitive control (Valian, 2014). These results confirm my hypothesis that specific aspects of bilingual advantage are strongly associated with specific bilingual experiences (L2 proficiency differences, interpreting experience, and public speaking experience). Some previous studies fail to capture the existence of bilingual advantage because of their not taking into account the differences existing among bilinguals as related to their language use experience.

Taken together, all these results answer the four specific questions and one general question raised above. The results of the experiments included in this volume support the existence of bilingual advantage and further clarify the relationship between specific aspects of bilingual experiences and specific aspects of cognitive control. In the following section, I will further discuss the findings with respect to the relationship between specific bilingual experience and specific aspects of cognitive control.

Table 18. A summary of the results in the current research.

Experiment 1		*Mono*	*Bili-0*	*Intpr-1*	*Intpr-2*	*Bili-1*	*Spk-1*	*Bili-2*	*Spk-2*
	L2 Proficiency	**-**						++	
	Interpreting	**-**						**-**	
	Public speaking	**-**						**-**	
Flanker	Congruent trial	**a**						**a**	
	Neutral trial	**a**						**a**	
	Incongruent trial	**a**						**a**	
	Conflict effect	**a**						**a**	
Number Stroop	Congruent trial	**a**						**a**	
	Neutral trial	**a**						**a**	
	Incongruent trial	**a**						**a**	
	Conflict effect	**a**						**a**	
WCST	Global RTs	**a**						**a**	
	Completed categories	**a**						**b**	
	Overall errors	**a**						**b**	
	Perseverative errors	**a**						**b**	
	Pre-category errors	**a**						**b**	
Experiment 2		*Mono*	*Bili-0*	*Intpr-1*	*Intpr-2*	*Bili-1*	*Spk-1*	*Bili-2*	*Spk-2*
	L2 Proficiency		+					++	
	Interpreting		**-**					**-**	
	Public speaking		**-**					**-**	
Flanker	Congruent trial		**a**					**a**	
	Neutral trial		**a**					**a**	
	Incongruent trial		**a**					**a**	
	Conflict effect		**a**					**a**	

Experiment 2		*Mono*	*Bili-0*	*Intpr-1*	*Intpr-2*	*Bili-1*	*Spk-1*	*Bili-2*	*Spk-2*
Number Stroop	Congruent trial		**a**					**a**	
	Neutral trial		**a**					**a**	
	Incongruent trial		**a**					**a**	
	Conflict effect		**a**					**a**	
WCST	Global RTs		**a**					**a**	
	Completed categories		**a**					**a**	
	Overall errors		**a**					**a**	
	Perseverative errors		**a**					**a**	
	Pre-category errors		**a**					**a**	
Experiment 3		*Mono*	*Bili-0*	*Intpr-1*	*Intpr-2*	*Bili-1*	*Spk-1*	*Bili-2*	*Spk-2*
	L2 Proficiency			++	+++	+		++	
	Interpreting			+	++	-		-	
	Public speaking			-	-	-		-	
Flanker	Congruent trial			**a**	**a**	**a**		**a**	
	Neutral trial			**a**	**a**	**a**		**a**	
	Incongruent trial			**a**	**a**	**a**		**a**	
	Conflict effect			**a**	**a**	**a**		**a**	
Number Stroop	Congruent trial			**a**	**a**	**a**		**a**	
	Neutral trial			**a**	**a**	**a**		**a**	
	Incongruent trial			**a**	**a**	**a**		**a**	
	Conflict effect			**a**	**a**	**a**		**a**	
WCST	Global RTs			**a**	**a**	**a**		**a**	
	Completed categories			**b**	**c**	**a**		**a**	
	Overall errors			**b**	**b**	**a**		**a**	
	Perseverative errors			**b**	**b**	**a**		**a**	
	Pre-category errors			**b**	**b**	**a**		**a**	

Experiment 4		Mono	Bili-0	Intpr-1	Intpr-2	Bili-1	Spk-1	Bili-2	Spk-2
	L2 Proficiency	-					+	++	++
	Interpreting	-					-	-	-
	Public speaking	-					+	-	+
Flanker	Congruent trial	**a**					**b**	**a**	**b**
	Neutral trial	**a**					**b**	**a**	**b**
	Incongruent trial	**a**					**b**	**a**	**b**
	Conflict effect	**a**					**a**	**a**	**a**
Number Stroop	Congruent trial	**a?**					**a?**	**a**	**b**
	Neutral trial	**a**					**a**	**a**	**b**
	Incongruent trial	/					**a**	**a**	**b**
	Conflict effect	**a**					**a**	**a**	**a**
WCST	Global RTs	**a**					**a**	**a**	**a**
	Completed categories	**a**					**a**	**b**	**b**
	Overall errors	**a**					**a**	**b**	**b**
	Perseverative errors	**a**					**a**	**b**	**b**
	Pre-category errors	**a**					**b**	**c**	**c**

Note: "Mono" means the monolingual group; "Bili" means the bilingual groups; "Intpr" means Interpreting groups; "Spk" means speaking groups; "-"means negative with particular experience, "+"means positive with particular experience, and "++" means more significant than "+" in degrees. Different letters "a, b, c" indicate that group differences are significant at $p<.05$ or $p<.01$ level. "**a**?" means significant at marginal level. "/" means insignificant compared with any group.

8.2 Bilingual Experiences and Aspects of Cognitive Control

In the current research, three aspects of bilingual advantage in cognitive control have been measured: *inhibition, conflict monitoring* and *mental set shifting*, which are actually the most commonly investigated subcomponents of cognitive control that have been reported related to bilingualism. Across the experiments in the current research, different aspects of bilingual advantage in cognitive control have been observed among different groups of bilinguals, who had distinctive bilingual experiences. Further discussion concerning the relationship between different bilingual experiences and different aspects of bilingual advantage in cognitive control will be presented in the following sections.

8.2.1 Bilingual Experiences and Inhibition

Previous studies regarding bilingual advantage started largely from the hypothesis that bilinguals are better at inhibition because they need to select goal-relevant information and inhibit competing and distracting information. Much of the work on bilingual advantage on inhibition (conflict resolution) is supported by Green's Inhibitory Control theory (1998). According to the theory, in bilingual language processing, both languages are activated. In order to retrieve the target language, bilinguals have to inhibit the non-target language lemmas. The long-term practice of such inhibitory control in language processing may transfer to general cognitive control in conflict resolution. If bilingual advantage exists, the conflict produced by incongruent trials could be expected to be larger for monolinguals than for bilinguals (Bialystok et al., 2008; Bialystok et al., 2004; Costa et al., 2008; Paap & Greenberg, 2013). The different RTs in congruent trials and incongruent trials of behavioral tasks such as the Flanker, the Simon, and the Stroop are usually taken to index the ability to suppress irrelevant information.

Previous studies examine the Simon interference effect and the Flanker interference effect (different RTs between congruent and incongruent trials). However, few experiments report large interference effect, particularly among young adults (Hilchey & Klein, 2011), but the effect seems to be more pronounced in middle-aged and old-aged bilinguals (Bialystok et al., 2004; Bialystok et al., 2005; see review by Bialystok et al., 2009).

In the current experiments, the Flanker task and the Number Stroop task were used to test the aspect of inhibition. The standard marker of inhibition is the difference in mean response times between trials that require conflict resolution and trials that do not in the two tasks. We find no difference between the monolinguals and the bilinguals or between different bilingual groups in the aspect of inhibition. In *Experiment One*, the young adult Chinese-English bilinguals do not differ from the Chinese monolinguals in either the Flanker conflict or the Number Stroop conflict. In *Experiment Two*, bilinguals differing in L2 proficiency do not show any difference in the Flanker conflict or the Number Stroop conflict. In *Experiment Three* and *Experiment Four*, bilinguals having interpreting experience and L1/L2 public speaking experience are not better than the control bilinguals and monolinguals in conflict resolution in either the Flanker task or the Number Stroop task.

These findings are not consistent with previous expectations by the Inhibitory Control theory, which states that bilinguals may be better at inhibition because they have intensive experience of inhibiting the non-target language representations in language processing. "Inhibition" may work through two processes (Green, 1998): firstly the intended goal is selected and the unintended goal is inhibited; secondly the lexical forms of relevant language are activated and the equivalents of the competing language are inhibited. If such intensive practice of language management or language control is related to a general ability, not specific to language, then bilinguals' cognitive control may be enhanced in the aspect of inhibiting interference in nonlinguistic tasks (Bialystok et al., 2009; Kroll & Bialystok, 2013; Paap & Greenberg, 2013), but the current experiments results provide no evidence of such advantage in inhibition.

However, the findings of the current research are consistent with a recent and comprehensive review of bilingual advantage, which concludes that evidence for a bilingual advantage in inhibitory control (inhibition) is rare in both children and young adults (Hilchey & Klein, 2011). Their review includes eight studies that adopt the standard Simon task to examine inhibitory control (inhibition) processes in bilinguals relative to monolinguals and four studies that employ the Flanker or ANT to investigate bilingual advantage. They conclude that few experiments report statistically significant bilingual advantage in inhibition, with the remaining data showing much smaller or little or no such bilingual advantage. The null effect on inhibition is also consistent with some more recent studies that observe no behavioral bilingual advantage, particularly among young-adult bilinguals (e.g., Paap & Greenberg, 2013; Gathercole et al., 2014).

Why is it that bilingual advantage in the aspect of inhibition in cognitive control is not observable? That the magnitude of conflict resolution (i.e., inhibition) is not easy to detect may be caused by the ratio of congruent trials to incongruent trials. If a task involves too few conflict monitoring resources, bilingual advantage in the magnitude of the conflict effect may not be detectable because the conflict resolution is either too easy (the majority of the trials are incongruent) or too difficult (the majority of the trials are congruent), and hence the effects of bilingualism upon inhibition may become undetectable (Costa et al., 2009).

However, this explanation is not confirmed yet. The conflict effect has received much attention, but it appears not to be reliable and robust. Some scholars have already questioned its usefulness to draw a strong conclusion regarding bilingual advantage (Colzato et al., 2008). Although our results add evidence to this concern, it is still reasonable to infer that some kind of inhibitory control is needed for preventing massive interference from the non-target language when the target language schema is activated. For example, in lexical selection, inhibition is involved to reduce competition between two lexical activations, which has been supported by both behavioral and electrophysiological evidence (Shao, Roelofs, Acheson, & Meyer, 2014), but in other situations such as interpreting, there may be no need for such intensive inhibition (Yudes et al., 2011).

Another possible explanation opposing the view mentioned in the literature review comes from the hypothesis that inhibition is common to all cognitive control and not specific to any subcomponent (Miyake & Friedman, 2012), thus not easy to isolate and detect its effect. In their view, each cognitive control construct can be divided into common cognitive control (unity) or specific ability control (diversity). By adopting the latent variable approach in examining the three components of inhibition, shifting, and updating, they conclude that, after accounting for the common variance for inhibition, there is no specific inhibition factor left. That is, inhibition correlates perfectly with cognitive control unity, but leaves no inhibition-specific variance.

Furthermore, these results are only based on behavioral tests, so they do not necessarily indicate null effect in other types of measurement, such as in ERPs or fMRI tests. It has been shown, for example, that after second-language training, bilinguals show larger P3 amplitude on the go–Nogo task and smaller P600 amplitude on the judgment task, indicating enhanced cognitive control in inhibition, with no changes for the control group and no differences between groups on behavioral measures (Sullivan et al., 2014). However, one thing worth noting is that the brain network differences measured by ERPs or fMRI between monolinguals and bilinguals or between different types of bilinguals only provide data showing that different groups react differently on brain network activations but do not directly tell whether or not it is advantageous or disadvantageous in terms of behavioral measures.

Therefore, it is more reasonable to suggest that bilingual advantage in inhibition (conflict resolution) may be limited to some conditions, for example, a particular language use experience in a given context where inhibition is intensively required. In other words, the nature of bilingual experience may influence the type of bilingual advantage observed (Tao et al., 2011). Future research is required to further examine the relationship between specific aspects of bilingual experience with inhibition in cognitive control.

8.2.2 Public Speaking Experience and Conflict Monitoring

Monitoring one's performance, internal states, and on-going context is another aspect of cognitive control in response to changing goals and mixing information. Although most previous studies focus on inhibition, some scholars have noticed that bilingual advantage may also exist in the ability to manage a complex set of rapidly changing task demands (Bialystok et al., 2004). In the current experiments, the standard marker of conflict monitoring is the overall response times of each trial type in the Flanker task and the Number Stroop task. Shorter overall RTs of each trial type (or condition) indicate a better/faster efficiency of conflict monitoring.

In the current experiments, we found significant evidence revealing that a particular group of bilinguals outperformed monolinguals or control bilinguals in the aspect of conflict monitoring, but limited only in situations for bilinguals with L2/L1 public speaking experience. In *Experiment One*, we compared general bilinguals and general monolinguals and found that the bilinguals did not outperform the monolinguals in overall RTs of different trial types in the Flanker task and the Number Stroop task. In *Experiment Two*, bilinguals differing in L2 proficiency did not show difference in overall RTs of different trial types in the same tasks. In *Experiment Three*, bilinguals with intensive interpreting experience did not outperform the control bilinguals in overall RTs of different trial types, suggesting that language interpreting experience does not significantly contribute to conflict monitoring in cognitive control. However, in *Experiment Four*, bilinguals with public speaking experience (particularly L2 public speaking) performed significantly faster than the control bilinguals and monolinguals in overall RTs of different trial types in the Flanker task. Moreover, bilinguals with L2 public speaking experience performed faster than L1 public speaking bilinguals, the control bilinguals, and the monolinguals in the Number Stroop task. These results indicate that public speaking experience, esp. in L2, contributes most significantly to the enhancement of conflict monitoring in cognitive control.

The superior ability of conflict monitoring for the public speaking bilinguals may come from the specific experience of public speaking itself. In public speaking, either in L1 or in L2, the speakers need to continuously monitor the appropriate context of language use, and then to attentively focus on the target language. Once the target language is selected, there is no need to change to another language, and there is no need to inhibit the non-target language since the non-target language is kept at a stable and low activation level. All these specific contexts may lead to a speedup of the overall RTs. Therefore, without continuously changing to the different demands associated to different types of trials, there is likely no enhancement of conflict resolution (Costa et al., 2009). Similarly, it is also reasonable to suspect that public speaking experience does not significantly contribute to differences in mental set shifting because there is no intensive need to switch between two languages in public speaking.

Costa et al. (2009) have discussed the origin of bilingual advantage in conflict monitoring. They suggest that bilingual advantage in overall RTs may reflect the ability to handle tasks that involve mixing trials of different types. Bilinguals may be faster going back and forth between trials that require conflict resolution and those without conflict (Costa et al., 2009). This may be caused by the fact that bilinguals need to continuously monitor what is appropriate for the current situation, which may include the target language, appropriateness of language production, interlocutor's knowledge and background. This global RTs advantage is somewhat unanticipated, and is beyond the sphere of the inhibitory control model and thus lacking a stable theoretical foundation (Hilchey & Klein, 2011).

However, more recent studies include monitoring as one important aspect/component of cognitive control related to bilingual advantage (Paap & Greenberg, 2013) or consider conflict monitoring to be one essential part of control processes to maintain a current goal (Green & Abutalebi, 2013).

The results in the current studies are also consistent with Hilchey and Klein (2011)'s review that bilingual advantage in conflict resolution/inhibitory control is scarce and usually absent, but bilinguals typically outperform monolinguals both in compatible and incompatible trials. The results also add new evidence to bilingual advantage in conflict monitoring, but the effect is detectable only for bilinguals with public speaking experience (particularly L2 public speaking). This suggests that only specific bilingual experience, rather than general bilingual learning, may significantly contribute to bilingual advantage in conflict monitoring. In some recent studies, the global RTs advantage has not been observed when examining bilinguals' performance in tasks such as the Flanker, the Simon, or the Stroop (e.g., Humphrey & Valian, 2012; Kousaie & Phillips, 2012b; Paap & Greenberg, 2013). The reasons may lie in the fact that they do not understand the specificity of language experience to be a crucial factor affecting cognitive control.

However, even though there is no group difference in the aspect of conflict monitoring in behavioral measures, it does not mean that there is no difference in electrophysiological measures. More and more recent studies are now adopting the ERPs technique to investigate this issue. For example, Rodriguez-Pujadas et al. (2014) test the hypothesis that early bilinguals and monolinguals use different brain areas when performing non-linguistic cognitive control tasks. They find that monolinguals activate the anterior cingulate cortex (ACC) more than bilinguals when performing the stop-signal task. These results offer direct support for the notion that bilinguals use the anterior cingulate more efficiently than monolinguals to monitor nonlinguistic cognitive conflicts, providing the precondition for behavioral advantages.

Based on the behavioral data from the current experiments, we cannot conclude that bilinguals are not superior to monolinguals in conflict monitoring, but we can conclude that bilinguals with public speaking experience really do enjoy stronger ability in conflict monitoring than bilinguals without such experience and monolinguals. Realistically, future studies in the field should establish a theory that links specific aspects of bilingual experience to specific aspects of cognitive control, perhaps referring to the adaptive control hypothesis proposed recently by Green and Abutalebi (2013).

8.2.3 L2 Proficiency, Language Interpreting, and Mental Set Shifting

Mental set shifting is a cognitive control function that concerns shifting back and forth between multiple tasks, operations, or mental sets (Monsell, 1996). It is also referred to as attention switching, or task switching. Shifting processes involves the disengagement of an irrelevant task set and the subsequent active engagement of a relevant task set (Miyake et al., 2000). Bilinguals are assumed to have a better ability in mental set shifting than monolinguals because they possess specific experience in switching from one language to the other. As both languages are activated in a bilingual mind, continual switching requires bilinguals to inhibit the lexical or syntactic equivalents of the non-target language and flexibly change into the other task set (language). In the current research, the WCST was used to measure the ability of mental set shifting. A better performance of the task indicates a superior ability of mental set shifting.

In the current experiments, we find that bilinguals have better ability in mental set shifting than monolinguals and that bilinguals with interpreting experience have better ability in mental set shifting as compared with bilinguals without such experience. In *Experiment One*, a group of bilinguals was compared with a group of monolinguals. The results show that the two groups did not differ in the tasks of Flanker and Number Stroop, but they differed significantly in the WCST task. This result provides support for the existence of bilingual advantage in mental set shifting. In *Experiment Two*, between two bilingual groups differing in L2 proficiency, no mental set shifting advantage was found for the higher L2 proficiency group. In *Experiment Three*, two bilingual groups differing in interpreting experience and L2 proficiency were compared with two bilingual groups without interpreting experience but differing in L2 proficiency. The results show that bilinguals with interpreting experience performed significantly better than the control bilinguals in the WCST task but not in the Flanker or Number Stroop tasks. Moreover, the bilingual group with a longer time of interpreting training (3 years) outperformed the bilingual group with a shorter time of interpreting training (1 year) after L2 proficiency was matched. In *Experiment Four*, the public speaking groups did not outperform the control bilingual groups or monolingual group in the WCST task, but the bilinguals with higher L2 proficiency performed better than bilinguals (or monolinguals) with lower L2 proficiency in the WCST task. The results from the four experiments are significant in many ways.

Firstly, these results suggest that bilingualism does contribute significantly to mental set shifting (as in *Experiment One*), which is consistent with some previous studies that provide explanations of such bilingual advantage. Peal and Lambert (1962) were the first to find that bilingual children are superior to their monolingual counterparts in symbol manipulation and reorganization. They suggest that bilinguals show better mental flexibility perhaps as a consequence of having to switch between their two languages. Moreover, in the following years, only a few studies further examined such shifting advantage, or suggested a relationship between bilingualism and mental set shifting in cognitive control (Bialystok & Martin, 2004; Festman & Munte, 2012; Linck, Schwieter, & Sunderman, 2011; Prior & Macwhinney, 2010; Rodriguez-Fornells et al., 2011; Soveri et al., 2011). The current research provides further evidence for the existence of bilingual advantage in mental set shifting, whereas most previous studies are concerned with bilingual advantage in inhibitory control.

Secondly, bilinguals with a higher L2 proficiency have better ability in mental set shifting. This result seems contradictory to the findings in *Experiment Two* and *Experiment Three*, in which no differences were found between bilingual groups differing in L2 proficiency. This can be explained by the fact that in *Experiment Four*, the magnitude of differences in L2 proficiency between the higher L2 proficiency group and the lower group was much greater than that between the bilingual groups in *Experiment Two* and *Experiment Three*. In *Experiment Two* and *Experiment Three*, all the subjects were English-majors and their difference in L2 proficiency was not practically great enough (19.5 vs. 23.2; 21.5 vs. 23.2) (although statistically significant), whereas the difference in L2 proficiency in *Experiment Four* between the four groups were significantly sharper (7.1 vs. 19.5 vs. 23.2 vs. 24.5). Additionally, in *Experiment Two* and *Experiment Three,* there was no monolingual control group, whereas in *Experiment Four,* the monolingual group was included for comparison. Moreover, in *Experiment Four,* the L1 public speaking group were non-English major students, whereas the L2 public speaking group and the bilingual group were English-major students. Distinct from *Experiment Two* and *Experiment Three*, *Experiment Four* included the bilingual or monolingual adults whose L2 proficiency was significantly more distinctive across groups. These sharper differences in L2 proficiency must have caused the performance differences in the WCST task that tested mental set shifting. Importantly enough, these results indicate that L2 proficiency contributes significantly to mental set shifting in cognitive control.

Thirdly, these results suggest that specific bilingual language-use experience such as language interpreting contributes more to mental set shifting since the experience intensifies the need to switch between two languages. As in the study conducted by Prior and Gollan (2011), a task switch (color and shape) paradigm was used. They find that good language switchers are also good task switchers (Prior & Gollan, 2011). Another recent study (Yudes et al., 2011) adopted the Wisconsin Card Sorting Test (WCST) to measure mental set shifting. A group of professional interpreters, a group of bilinguals and a group of monolinguals are compared. The results find that interpreters have a better ability in mental set shifting than their bilingual and the monolingual counterparts, but, out of expectation, there is no difference between bilinguals and monolinguals (Yudes et al., 2011). They explain that this might be caused by the fact that the participants were unbalanced bilinguals. However, the current research (*Experiment One)*, which also includes unbalanced (Chinese-English) bilinguals, provides robust evidence that bilinguals outperform monolinguals in mental set shifting. Furthermore, the current research (*Experiment Three*) shows that even bilinguals with interpreting experience (student interpreters rather than professional interpreters) perform significantly better than control bilinguals.

Fourthly, however, for the aspects of inhibition and conflict monitoring, the factors of L2 proficiency and language interpreting do not bring about group differences. We speculate that this is because neither L2 proficiency nor language interpreting engages participants in activities/practices requiring intensive demand to inhibit the non-target language when the target language is in use. As mentioned earlier, for interpreters there is no strong need for inhibition because both languages are kept at relatively high levels of activation for the convenience of continual mental set shifting (Yudes et al., 2011).

Together, the results from the current experiments and the results from previous literature consistently reveal that bilingualism does lead to the enhancement of mental set shifting in cognitive control and a significantly higher degree of bilingualism (i.e., by L2 proficiency) may contribute more to this enhancement. Moreover, more practice with language interpreting contributes more significantly to the enhancement of mental set shifting. All these findings suggest that the enhancement of mental set shifting, just as the aspect of conflict monitoring, is closely associated only with a certain specific bilingual experience. In future studies, more empirical work should be done and more experiment paradigms should be adopted to examine the aspect of mental set shifting in cognitive control, which is not much examined in previous literature.

The four experiments in this volume demonstrate a clear relationship between bilingual experiences in ecology and specific aspects of bilingual advantage in cognitive control. The results altogether suggest that the enhancement of specific aspects of cognitive control is closely associated with specific features of bilingual experience in behavioral ecology. The specific language experience of how bilinguals use their languages in a specific context, greatly affects which aspect of cognitive control is enhanced. This line of research may help clarify which facet of bilingualism genuinely contributes to specific aspect(s) of cognitive control advantage.

8.3 The Incoherence Problem

Previous studies demonstrate bilingual advantage in cognitive control for bilinguals relative to monolinguals. Bilingual advantage is observed in different aspects of cognitive control, including sometimes inhibitory control (inhibition) (at least claimed so), but other-times conflict monitoring and mental set shifting. However, bilingual advantage is not found consistently in all studies. Quite a few studies observe null effect of bilingual advantage, particularly among young-adult bilinguals. Moreover, even among the studies that observe bilingual advantage, there is no coherence across the tasks measuring the same construct of cognitive control (Paap & Greenberg, 2013).

However, the current research results reveal that bilingual advantage does exist, and different aspects of bilingual advantage are present only when different bilingual experiences are distinguished. By adopting multiple tasks measuring multiple aspects of cognitive control, we compared cognitive control differences between different bilingual groups who differed in bilingual language experiences. The results show that specific bilingual experience (i.e., L2 proficiency, interpreting, and public speaking) contributes distinctively to different aspects of cognitive control. Therefore, the observed "incoherence" problem of bilingual advantage may be caused by different factors, both theoretical and methodological.

First, bilingual experience is heterogeneous from different perspectives. Some are simultaneous bilinguals who learn two languages at the same time whereas others are sequential bilinguals who learn a second language after their native tongue has been acquired. Besides the external factors (which are external to bilingualism itself) such as age, cultural background, and individual differences, bilinguals vary greatly in terms of their bilingual experiences, such as their language proficiency, language interpreting, L2 speaking, and L2 reading abilities (Gold et al., 2013; Iluz-Cohen & Armon-Lotem, 2013; Singh & Mishra, 2012; Tao et al., 2011). These varieties in bilingual experience may cause a mixture of positive effect and null effect, both between bilinguals and monolinguals, and between different groups of bilinguals.

Second, the construct of cognitive control is diversified. According to previous literature, cognitive control can be decomposed into multiple aspects, including inhibition, mental set shifting, working memory updating, conflict monitoring, response control, and selective attention (Green & Abutalebi, 2013; Miller & Cohen, 2001; Miyake et al., 2000). We are not sure exactly how many subcomponents can be identified, but it is widely accepted that cognitive control can be separated into multiple aspects. This means that the enhancement of one aspect (i.e., *mental set shifting*) of cognitive control by bilingualism may not indicate the enhancement of another (i.e., *inhibition*). The diversity of the cognitive control construct is surely one significant factor confounding previous findings related to bilingual advantage.

Third, most of the evidence of bilingual advantage comes from studies using tasks such as the Simon task, the Flanker task, the Stroop task, the task switch, and the card sorting task etc., but not using them in a consistent way across different samples of bilinguals. Either one task is adopted in each study, or different single tasks are adopted in different studies. Therefore, it is not convenient to compare different bilingual groups and to compare different aspects of cognitive control.

Fourth, the comparison between bilinguals and monolinguals in bilingual advantage research highlights the theory that bilinguals have cognitive control advantage over monolinguals, but it does not tell us what about bilingualism causes this advantage.

These factors have been at least under-examined or largely ignored in previous research, thus leading to the seemingly "incoherence" problem of bilingual advantage. However, when all these factors are seriously taken into account, the current research presents a clearer picture of the nature of bilingual advantage. The experiments' results in the current research confirm the existence of bilingual advantage in specific aspects of cognitive control. Furthermore, the experiment results in the current research clarify the relationship between specific bilingual experience (L2 proficiency, language interpreting, and public speaking) and specific aspects of bilingual advantage in cognitive control (inhibition, conflict monitoring, and mental set shifting).

8.4 Summary

This chapter has discussed the results of the current research. More importantly, detailed and profound discussions have been presented to elaborate the possible relationship between different bilingual experiences and specific aspects of cognitive control. Finally, the chapter has presented how the "incoherence" problem of bilingual advantage in previous studies can be explained in the current research by some crucial factors, including the heterogeneity of bilingual experience and diversity of cognitive control.

Chapter 9: Conclusions and Implications

9.1 Major Findings of the Current Research

By comparing young adult Chinese-English bilinguals and counterpart Chinese monolinguals and by comparing different groups of young adult Chinese-English bilinguals who have distinctive bilingual experiences, the major findings of the current research are:

1) Bilingual advantage does exist among young adult Chinese-English bilinguals (but only in mental set shifting tested by the WCST);
2) L2 proficiency contributes significantly to the aspect of mental set shifting (tested by the WCST), rather than inhibition or conflict monitoring, in cognitive control, but only when L2 proficiency differences reach a certain level.
3) A certain degree of language interpreting experience significantly enhances the aspect of mental set shifting, rather than inhibition or conflict monitoring, in cognitive control (tested by the WCST);
4) A certain degree of public speaking experience, particularly L2 public speaking, significantly enhances the aspect of conflict monitoring, rather than inhibition or mental set shifting, in cognitive control (tested by the Flanker task and the Number Stroop task).

The research results from the four experiments answer the research questions and support my hypotheses in the volume. Based on the findings, it is reasonable to conclude that different bilingual experiences affect different aspects of bilingual advantage in cognitive control. It is of great importance to examine bilingual advantage by considering the two core concepts of the heterogeneity of bilingual experience (the nature of bilingualism) and the diversity of cognitive control (the nature of cognitive control). This line of investigation will significantly illuminate the nature of bilingual advantage.

9.2 Theoretical and Practical Implications

The interest in the investigation of bilingual advantage in cognitive control is growing. A large amount of studies show that bilingualism changes the neurocognitive mechanism, enhances cognitive control, and helps maintain a "cognitive reserve" for bilinguals.

Although the studies concerning bilingual advantage have not been fully included and bilingual advantage has not been fully characterized, the experiments concerned here in the current research have great *implications* in theory and add to the growing literature in this area and raise questions with respect to the robustness and generalizability of the suggested bilingual advantage.

Firstly, in the current research (*Experiment* One) of this dissertation, the comparison between monolinguals and bilinguals further supports the theory that bilingualism brings about cognitive control advantage. It is important to note that even among young adult bilinguals, who are at the peak of cognitive functioning, it is still possible for them to demonstrate advantages in cognitive control. And these advantages can also translate into behavioral differences. At least two aspects of the study of bilingual advantage are very different from previous studies. First, in *Experiment One*, the linguistic and cultural homogeneity of the bilinguals and monolinguals was manipulated, whereas in most previous studies, bilinguals had different first languages and cultural backgrounds. Second, *Experiment One* is one of the few to find bilingual advantage among young adult Chinese-English learners who have been learning English as a foreign language. This result will obviously add more to the generalization of the theory of bilingual advantage.

Secondly, the comparisons between different bilingual groups who have different bilingual experiences offer us a better window to examine which aspect of bilingualism contributes to bilingual advantage.

The results of different experiments in this volume show that different bilingual populations with different bilingual (language use) experiences display differences in cognitive control enhancement. It is important to note that this volume is one of the first to provide empirical evidence that bilingual cognitive control advantage is determined by how languages are used in behavioral ecology as few studies (e.g., Green, 2011; Valian, 2014) suggests the specificity of language use context in ecology. The lack of considering language use experiences as a highly significant contributor to bilingual advantage may be a factor confounding relevant research results in previous studies. More specifically, this volume is the first to identify the relationship between specific characteristics of bilingual experience in ecology and specific aspects of cognitive control. To illustrate, *Experiment Two* examines the limited role of L2 proficiency in predicting group difference in cognitive control among different groups of bilinguals. The results show that the role of L2 proficiency is not significant, but in *Experiment Four* when the L2 proficiency difference was greater, the effect is found for mental set shifting. Higher L2 proficiency brings about better ability of mental set shifting. *Experiment Three* and *Experiment Four*, by taking two specific typical language use examples, find that language use experience plays a crucial role in bilingual advantage. For the language interpreting groups, the bilinguals' cognitive control abilities are greatly enhanced in the aspect of mental set shifting, which is closely related to language switching experience. Meanwhile, for the public speaking groups (particularly L2 speaking), the bilinguals' cognitive control abilities are greatly enhanced in the aspect of conflict monitoring, which underlies the mechanism required in the experience of public speaking. All these results support the hypothesis that different bilingual experiences enhance different aspects of cognitive control.

Thirdly, these new findings clearly point to the nature of bilingual advantage and encourage further relevant studies in future. Numerous studies examine bilingual advantage between monolinguals and bilinguals. However, the concept of bilingual advantage remains unclear as few studies directly examine its specific origins. Moreover, as a term, bilingualism still remains a too general as it does not distinguish specific subcomponents. The incoherence of the findings concerning bilingual advantage in previous studies, particularly among young adults, leads us to conclude that within the big umbrella of "bilingual advantage", there are still varieties and heterogeneities. The results of the current research raise some important issues concerning bilingual advantage: i) bilingual advantage is present only in certain aspects of cognitive control, and these aspects of cognitive control are influenced by certain bilingual experience. For example, public speaking experience enhances conflict monitoring and language interpreting experience enhances mental set shifting; ii) traditional bilingual advantage in inhibition is present in very limited conditions, but, the advantage may be present more often in the aspects of conflict monitoring or mental set shifting. These issues are of great importance in that they clarify the nature of bilingual advantage and that they explain the incoherence problem of bilingual advantage observed recently in quite a few studies.

Green and Abutalebi (2013)'s adaptive control hypothesis supports the current results. As already mentioned in the introduction, eight processes (or sub-compositions) of cognitive control are identified: *goal maintenance, conflict monitoring, interference suppression, salient cue detection, selective response inhibition, task disengagement, task engagement, and opportunistic planning*. In the hypothesis, the processes of control themselves adapt to the demands placed upon them. It is the interactional context for the bilingual speakers that drives the adaptive response. When the bilingual interactional context varies, the demand on these control processes will change, thus resulting in variations of enhancement in general cognitive control. Three general interactional contexts are identified as these contexts reflect the everyday conversational use of language: single language, dual language, and dense code-switching. In a single language context, one language is used in one environment and the other in a second distinctive environment. For example, a bilingual child may speak his native language at home and the other at school. In such a context, there is no frequent language switching. In a dual language context, both languages are used, but with different speakers. For example, interpreters speak/switch two languages in a conversation but to different speakers. In a dense-code switching context, speakers interweave their two languages within a single utterance. For example, in English-Chinese dense-code switch, a typical utterance may be like this: "If you are free, can you song (drive) me?"

Relating the different interactional contexts with cognitive control processes, they hypothesize that the single language context may generally enhance the processes of goal maintenance, conflict monitoring and interference suppression, the dual language context may generally enhance all the 7 processes except opportunistic planning, and dense code-switching context may generally enhance opportunistic planning. These predictions may be not necessarily precise, but the perspective that these control processes vary as a function of the interactional context is profound and provocative. The results from the current experiments are generally consistent with this hypothesis. Moreover, we have extended the context to more specific situations such as in interpreting and public speaking contexts. Exploration of the adaptive control hypothesis requires a continued effort to examine the relationship between specific patterns of interactional contexts and specific aspects of cognitive control, which would be best detected by a range of cognitive control tasks.

Besides theoretical implications, this volume has also significant *implications* in methodological practice.

Firstly, the research of bilingual advantage in the current volume is not limited to studies comparing bilinguals and monolinguals. Comparisons only between bilinguals and monolinguals do not offer us a way to sort out specific and fundamental origins of bilingual advantage, but comparisons between bilinguals of different groups with differing characteristics can do so. Most previous studies use independent samples of bilinguals and monolinguals to investigate bilingual advantage, but this method does not clarify which specific aspects of bilingualism fundamentally contribute to bilingual advantage.

Secondly, most previous studies use one independent task to examine bilingual advantage for each study, thus making it difficult to compare the results cross different participant groups, even though the tasks adopted are more or less similar. In the current volume, the same three tasks of Flanker, Number Stroop and WCST are used consistently across all the four experiments, thus providing us a good chance to compare the way in which language use experiences may have effects on different aspects of cognitive control. This is also helpful for us to identify the reliability of bilingual advantage in similar cross-task measurements.

Combined with the current research results, the literature works show that bilingual advantage exists among different bilinguals groups, including children, young adults, and mid-old age bilinguals. These conclusions have *implications* also for research concerning deficit cognitive control populations.

Firstly, numerous studies report that child bilinguals outperform their counterpart monolinguals in cognitive control when performing executive tasks such as the Simon task, the card sorting task etc. (Bialystok & Martin, 2004; Bialystok et al., 2005). The facilitative benefits in cognitive control brought about by bilingualism have implications in children's bilingual education. They provide a possible framework for designing bilingual education policy, teaching syllabus, and cognition-based bilingual learning.

Secondly, there are also abundant reports indicating that bilingualism delays the onset of Alzheimer's disease in old adult bilinguals (Bialystok et al., 2007; Bialystok et al., 2005; Gold et al., 2013) because the experience of a lifelong bilingualism provides a form of "cognitive reserve" that protects against age-related cognitive decline (Bialystok et al., 2004; Craik et al., 2010; Kave, Eyal, Shorek, & Cohen-Mansfield, 2008; Schweizer et al., 2012). Therefore, providing and promoting bilingual education and achieving a fluency of a second language, may offer a preventative measure against dementia for aging seniors. This bilingual language therapy is very practical and useful and it is also a possible way to increase the general quality of life in a given population, since there are more and more older adults in our society.

Thirdly, as our results show, bilingual advantage is evident even among young adult unbalanced Chinese-English bilinguals, and specific aspects of cognitive control can be enhanced as a result of specific intensive language use experiences. These results of bilingual advantage provide us with a new perspective of the relationship between bilingualism and cognitive control. If language control enhancement transfers to general cognitive control, it may also be true in the other direction. Therefore, the enhancement of general cognitive control might also be transferred to better language control, thus facilitating bilingual language learning/processing. There are already some studies or suggestions persisting to this theme (Gao, 2009; Hussey & Novick, 2012; Linck et al., 2011; Millner, Jaroszewski, Chamarthi, & Pizzagalli, 2012).

9.3 Limitations

Although the current experiments' results are of great significance for the study of bilingual advantage and for the relationship between specific aspects of bilingual experience and specific aspects of cognitive control, there are some limitations, which are common to all the four experiments in the current research.

Firstly, in recruiting the participants, our bilingual subjects were only limited to English learners who took English as a foreign language. It may be that Chinese-English bilinguals usually use the second language in class or for learning purposes and they do not use English as frequently as those immigrants in America or in other bilingual areas. Therefore, the research in this volume does not concern bilinguals who use their languages in family contexts and outside of academic learning.

Secondly, although all our participants came from similar family backgrounds, we did not include an objective test of SES, which is reported to be a possible factor affecting cognitive control. Therefore, a more objective measure of SES is necessary in future studies.

Thirdly, the absence of behavioral differences does not absolutely mean that cognitive processing differences do not exist between monolinguals and bilinguals or between different groups of bilinguals. Besides behavioral tools, future studies may adopt ERPs and fMRI techniques for complement. Even if no effect is found in behavioral measures, it is still necessary for us to know the potential differences in the neural correlates of cognitive control performance between monolinguals and bilinguals and between different types of bilinguals. Although a few behavioral studies detect bilingual advantage in inhibition by similar tasks (Bialystok et al., 2004; Bialystok et al., 2006; Carlson & Meltzoff, 2008), the current experiments find no group difference between the experiment group(s) and the control group(s). However, the null effect in behavioral measures observed in the current experiments does not fundamentally rule out the possibility of bilingual advantage in this aspect. If measured by ERPs or fMRI techniques, it is possible that bilingual advantage can be observed in neural activities.

Finally, only three main aspects of cognitive control (*inhibition, conflict monitoring, and mental set shifting*) are examined; it is possible that bilingualism incurs cognitive control advantage in other aspects. Future studies should design appropriate paradigms to test other possible aspects of bilingual advantage in cognitive control.

9.4 Future Directions

Based on the research results and the limitations in the current research, some future research directions relevant to bilingual advantage are proposed.

Firstly, future research is required to further clarify the role of L2 proficiency and the effect of inhibition in bilingual advantage by adopting ERPs or fMRI techniques. No cognitive control difference is observed between bilinguals of differing L2 proficiency in *Experiment Two* and *Experiment Three* where L2 learning background is controlled. And no effect of bilingual advantage in *inhibition* is detected across all the four experiments. However, the absence of bilingual advantage in behavioral results does not indicate the lack of difference in electrophysiological measurements.

Secondly, a more practical standard/degree of bilingualism (rather than statistical difference) needs to be advanced in order to achieve a clear understanding of what degree of bilingualism is prerequisite for bilingual advantage to manifest itself in cognitive control.

Thirdly, relevant to the nuclear research topic in this volume, more typical examples of bilingual language use patterns need to be identified so as to find out how a particular pattern of bilingual language use experience affects cognitive control.

Fourthly, the construct of cognitive control is both unitary and diversified. The aspects of inhibition, conflict monitoring, and mental set shifting, as tested in the current research, are just some main components of the general cognitive control construct. This suggests that there are other aspects that have not been identified yet, so future study should explore bilingual advantage in other aspects/components of cognitive control.

Finally, cognitive improvement for bilinguals may not be confined only to the construct of "control". It is reported that bilingualism has cognitive benefits in various aspects, apart from cognitive control. For example, there are already studies indicating that bilingual children have a better perspective-taking ability compared with monolinguals, extending bilingual advantage in cognitive control to spatial reasoning (Brown-Schmidt, 2009; Greenberg, Bellana, & Bialystok, 2013). Future studies may extend to a wider scope of investigation such as to metalinguistic awareness (Bialystok et al., 2012), language ambiguity (Dewaele & Wei, 2012), creativeness (Hommel et al., 2011; Kharkhurin, 2011; Leikin, 2012), reasoning about other people's beliefs (Rubio-Fernández & Glucksberg, 2012) and so on.

To highlight, it is very important to acknowledge that bilinguals are of different types. Identifying the types or patterns of how they use their languages and clarifying their respective relationships with specific aspects of cognitive control should be priorities in future studies. In addition, more sensitive measuring techniques such as ERPs or fMRI may be more suitable for measuring bilingual advantage when behavioral differences are absent. To conclude, the findings reported in the current research have both theoretical and practical implications in general cognitive research, cognitive control, as well as in future research examining children's cognitive development, learners' cognitive training, older adults' cognitive reserve, and other cognitive areas such as in reasoning and creativity.

References

Abutalebi, & Green. (2007). Bilingual language production: The neurocognition of language representation and control. *Journal of Neurolinguistics, 20*(3), 242–275.

Abutalebi, & Green. (2008). Control mechanisms in bilingual language production: Neural evidence from language switching studies. *Language and Cognitive Processes, 23*(4), 557–582.

Abutalebi, J. (2008). Neural aspects of second language representation and language control. *Acta Psychologica (Amst), 128*(3), 466–478.

Abutalebi, J., Annoni, J. M., Zimine, I., Pegna, A. J., Seghier, M. L., Lee-Jahnke, H., … Khateb, A. (2008). Language control and lexical competition in bilinguals: an event-related FMRI study. *Cerebral Cortex, 18*(7), 1496–1505.

Abutalebi, J., Della Rosa, P. A., Ding, G., Weekes, B., Costa, A., & Green, D. W. (2013). Language proficiency modulates the engagement of cognitive control areas in multilinguals. *Cortex, 49*(3), 905–911.

Abutalebi, J., Della Rosa, P. A., Green, D. W., Hernandez, M., Scifo, P., Keim, R., … Costa, A. (2012). Bilingualism tunes the anterior cingulate cortex for conflict monitoring. *Cerebral Cortex, 22*(9), 2076–2086.

Anderson, P. J. (2002). Assessment and development of executive functioning (EF) in childhood. *Child Neuropsychology, 8*(2), 71–82.

Anderson, V. A., Anderson, P., Northan, E., Jacobs, R., & Catroppa, C. (2001). Development of executive functions through late childhood and adolescence in an Australian sample. *Developmental Neuropsychology, 20*(1), 385–406.

Anton, E., Dunabeitia, J. A., Estevez, A., Hernandez, J. A., Castillo, A., Fuentes, L. J., … Carreiras, M. (2014). Is there a bilingual advantage in the ANT task? Evidence from children. *Frontiers in Psychology, 5*, 398. doi: 10.3389/fpsyg.2014.00398.

Appelbaum, L. G., Meyerhoff, K. L., & Woldorff, M. G. (2009). Priming and backward influences in the human brain: Processing interactions during the Stroop interference effect. *Cerebral Cortex, 19*(11), 2508–2521.

Ardal, S., Donald, M. W., Meuter, R., Muldrew, S., & Luce, M. (1990). Brain responses to semantic incongruity in bilinguals. *Brain and Language, 39*(2), 187–205.

Aron, A. R. (2007). The neural basis of inhibition in cognitive control. *Neuroscientist, 13*(3), 214–228.

Baddeley, A. D. (1986). *Working memory*. Oxford: Clarendon Press.

Barac, R., & Bialystok, E. (2012). Bilingual effects on cognitive and linguistic development: role of language, cultural background, and education. *Child Development, 83*(2), 413–422.

Barac, R., Bialystok, E., Castro, D. C., & Sanchez, M. (2014). The cognitive development of young dual language learners: A critical review. *Early Childhood Research Quarterly*. 29(4), 699–714.

Barceló, F., & Knight, R. T. (2002). Both random and perseverative errors underlie WCST deficits in prefrontal patients. *Neuropsychologia, 40*(3), 349–356.

Barkley, R. A. (1997). Behavioral inhibition, sustained attention, and executive functions: Constructing a unifying theory of ADHD. *Psychological Bulletin, 121*(1), 65–94.

Barry, D., & Petry, N. M. (2008). Predictors of decision-making on the Iowa Gambling Task: Independent effects of life time history of substance use disorders and performance on the Trail MakingTest. *Brain and Cognition, 66*, 243–252.

Bartolotti, J., & Marian, V. (2012). Language learning and control in monolinguals and bilinguals. *Cognitive Science, 36*(6), 1129–1147.

Beauvillain, C., & Grainger, J. (1987). Accessing lnterlexical Homographs: Some Limitations of a Language-Selective Access *Journal of Memory and Language, 26*, 658–672.

Ben-Zeev, S. (1977). The influence of bilingualism on cognitive strategy and cognitive development. *Child Development, 48*, 1009–1018.

Bergamaschi, M. M., Queiroz, R. H., Chagas, M. H., de Oliveira, D. C., De Martinis, B. S., Kapczinski, F., … Crippa, J. A. (2011). Cannabidiol reduces the anxiety induced by simulated public speaking in treatment-naive social phobia patients. *Neuropsychopharmacology, 36*(6), 1219–1226.

Best, J. R., Miller, P. H., & Jones, L. L. (2009). Executive functions after age 5: Changes and correlates. *Developmental Review, 29*(3), 180–200.

Bialystok. (1986). Factors in the growth of linguistic awareness. *Child Development, 57*, 498–510.

Bialystok, Peets, Moreno, & Sylvain. (2012). Producing bilinguals through immersion education: Development of metalinguistic awareness. *Applied Psycholinguistics*, 35(1), 177–191.

Bialystok, E. (1987). Influences of bilingualism on metalinguistic development. *Second Language Research, 3*(2), 154–166.

Bialystok, E. (1999). Cognitive complexity and attentional control in the bilingual mind. *Child Development, 70*, 636–644.

Bialystok, E. (2001). Metalinguistic aspects of bilingual processing. *Annual Review of Applied Linguistics, 21*, 169–181.

Bialystok, E. (2009). Bilingualism: The good, the bad, and the indifferent. *Bilingualism: Language and Cognition, 12*(01), 3–11.

Bialystok, E. (2010). Global-local and trail-making tasks by monolingual and bilingual children: beyond inhibition. *Developmental Psychology, 46*(1), 93–105.

Bialystok, E. (2011). Reshaping the mind: the benefits of bilingualism. *Canadian journal of experimental psychology, 65*(4), 229–235.

Bialystok, E., Barac, R., Blaye, A., & Poulin-Dubois, D. (2010). Word Mapping and Executive Functioning in Young Monolingual and Bilingual Children. *Journal of Cognition and Development, 11*(4), 485–508.

Bialystok, E., Craik, F. I. M., & Freedman, M. (2007). Bilingualism as a protection against the onset of symptoms of dementia. *Neuropsychologia, 45*(2), 459–464.

Bialystok, E., Craik, F. I. M., Grady, C., Chau, W., Ishii, R., Gunji, A., & Pantev, C. (2005). Effect of bilingualism on cognitive control in the Simon task: evidence from MEG. *Neuroimage, 24*(1), 40–49.

Bialystok, E., Craik, F. I. M., Green, D. W., & Gollan, T. H. (2009). Bilingual Minds. *Psychological Science in the Public Interest, 10*(3), 89–129.

Bialystok, E., Craik, F. I.M., Klein, R., & Viswanathan, M. (2004). Bilingualism, aging, and cognitive control: evidence from the Simon task. *Psychology and Aging, 19*(2), 290–303.

Bialystok, E., Craik, F. I. M., & Luk, G. (2008). Lexical access in bilinguals: Effects of vocabulary size and executive control. *Journal of Neurolinguistics, 21*(6), 522–538.

Bialystok, E., Craik, F. I. M., & Luk, G. (2012). Bilingualism: consequences for mind and brain. *Trends in Cognitive Sciences, 16*(4), 240–250.

Bialystok, E., Craik, F. I. M., & Ryan, J. (2006). Executive Control in a Modified Antisaccade Task: Effects of Aging and Bilingualism. *Journal of Experimental Psychology: Learning, Memory, and Cognition, 32*(6), 1341–1354.

Bialystok, E., Luk, G., Peets, K. F., & Yang, S. (2010). Receptive vocabulary differences in monolingual and bilingual children. *Bilingualism: Language and Cognition, 13*(04), 525–531.

Bialystok, E., & Martin, M. M. (2004). Attention and inhibition in bilingual children: evidence from the dimensional change card sort task. *Developmental Science 7*(3), 325–339.

Bialystok, E., Martin, M. M., & Viswanathan, M. (2005). Bilingualism across the lifespan: The rise and fall of inhibitory control. *International Journal of Bilingualism, 9*(1), 103–119.

Bialystok, E., & Viswanathan, M. (2009). Components of executive control with advantages for bilingual children in two cultures. *Cognition, 112*(3), 494–500.

Blumenfeld, H. K., & Marian, V. (2007). Constraints on parallel activation in bilingual spoken language processing: Examining proficiency and lexical status using eye-tracking. *Language and Cognitive Processes, 22*(5), 633–660.

Bradley, K. A. L., King, K. E., & Hernandez, A. E. (2012). Language experience differentiates prefrontal and subcortical activation of the cognitive control network in novel word learning. *Neuroimage, 67C*, 101–110.

Brocki, K. C., & Bohlin, G. (2004). Executive functions in children aged 6 to 13: A dimensional and developmental study. *Developmental Neuropsychology, 26*(2), 571–593.

Brown-Schmidt, S. (2009). The role of executive function in perspective taking during online language comprehension. *Psychonomic Bulletin and Review, 16*(5), 893–900.

Bush, G., Whalen, P. J., Rosen, B. R., Jenike, M. A., McInerney, S. C., & Rauch, S. L. (1998). The Counting Stroop: An Interference Task Specialized for Functional Neuroimaging – Validation Study With Functiona lMRI. *Human Brain Mapping, 6*, 270–282.

Carlson, S. M., & Meltzoff, A. N. (2008). Bilingual experience and executive functioning in young children. *Developmental Science, 11*(2), 282–298.

Christoffels, Kroll, & Bajo. (2013). Introduction to Bilingualism and Cognitive Control. *Frontiers in Psychology, 4*, 1–3. doi: 10.3389/fpsyg.2013.00199.

Coderre, E. L. (2012). Exploring the cognitive effects of bilingualism: neuroimaging investigations of lexical processing executive control, and the bilingual advantage. Doctor of Philosophy, University of Nottingham.

Colomé, À. (2001). Lexical Activation in Bilinguals' Speech Production: Language-Specific or Language-Independent? *Journal of Memory and Language, 45*(4), 721–736.

Colzato, L. S., Bajo, M. T., van den Wildenberg, W., Paolieri, D., Nieuwenhuis, S., La Heij, W., & Hommel, B. (2008). How does bilingualism improve executive control? A comparison of active and reactive inhibition mechanisms. *Journal of Experimental Psychology: Learning, Memory, and Cognition, 34*(2), 302–312.

Costa ,A.,&Caramazza,A.(1999). Is lexical selection in bilingual speech production languagespecific? Further evidence from Spanish-English and English-Spanish bilinguals. *Bilingualism: Language and Cognition, 2*(03), 231–244.

Costa, A., Caramazza, A., & Sebastian-Galles, N. (2000). The Cognate Facilitation Effect: Implications for Models of Lexical Access. *Journal of Experimental Psychology: Learning, Memory, and Cognition, 26*(5), 1283–1296.

Costa, A., Hernandez, M., Costa-Faidella, J., & Sebastian-Galles, N. (2009). On the bilingual advantage in conflict processing: now you see it, now you don't. *Cognition, 113*(2), 135–149.

Costa, A., Hernandez, M., & Sebastian-Galles, N. (2008). Bilingualism aids conflict resolution: evidence from the ANT task. *Cognition, 106*(1), 59–86.
Costa, A., Miozzo, M., & Caramazza, A. (1999). Lexical Selection in Bilinguals: Do Words in the Bilingual's Two Lexicons Compete for Selection? *Journal of Memory and Language, 41*, 365–397.
Costa, A., Santesteban, M., & Ivanova, I. (2006). How do highly proficient bilinguals control their lexicalization process? Inhibitory and language-specific selection mechanisms are both functional. *Journal of Experimental Psychology: Learning, Memory, and Cognition, 32*(5), 1057–1074.
Craik, F. I., Bialystok, E., & Freedman, M. (2010). Delaying the onset of Alzheimer disease: bilingualism as a form of cognitive reserve. *Neurology, 75*(19), 1726–1729.
Cummins, J. (1978). Bilingualism and the Development of Metalinguistic Awareness. *Psychology Journal of Cross-Cultural Psychology, 9*, 131–149.
Davidson, D. J., & Indefrey, P. (2011). Error-related activity and correlates of grammatical plasticity. *Frontiers in Psychology, 2*, 219. doi: 10.3389/fpsyg.2011.00219.
De Groot, A. M. B., Delmaar, P., & Lupker, S. J. (2000). The processing of interlexical homographs in translation recognition and lexical decision:Support for non-selective access to bilingual memory. *The Quarterly Journal of Experimental Psychology, 53A (2)*, 397–428.
De Bot, K. (1992). A bilingual production model: Levelt's "speaking" model adapted. *Applied Linguistics, 13*, 1–24.
De Bruijn, R. A., Dijkstra, T., Chwilla, D. J., & Schriefers, H. J. (2001). Language context affects on interlingual homograph recognition: evidence from event-related potentials and response times in semantic priming. *Bilingual Language Cognition, 4*, 155–168.
De Groot, & Christoffels. (2006). Language control in bilinguals: Monolingual tasks and simultaneous interpreting. *Bilingualism: Language and Cognition, 9*(2), 189–201.
De Luca, C. R., & Leventer, R. J. (2008). Developmental trajectories of executive functions across the lifespan. In P. Anderson, V. Anderson & R. Jacobs (Eds.), *Executive functions and the*

frontal lobes: a lifespan perspective (pp. 3–21). Washington, DC: Taylor & Francis.

De Luca, C. R., Wood, S. J., Anderson, V., Buchanan, J. A., Proffitt, T., Mahoney, K., & Panteli, C. (2003). Normative data from the CANTAB I: Development of executive function over the lifespan. *Journal of Clinical and Experimental Neuropsychology*, 242–254.

De Moor, W. (1998). *Visual word recognition in bilinguals.* Master thesis, University of Ghent, unpublished.

Dewaele, J.-M., & Wei, L. I. (2012). Is multilingualism linked to a higher tolerance of ambiguity? *Bilingualism: Language and Cognition, 16*(01), 231–240.

Dijkstra, T., & van Heuven, W. J. B. (1998). The BIA-model and bilingual word recognition. In J. Grainger & A. Jacobs (Eds.), *Localist connectionistic approaches to human cognition*. Mahaw, NJ: Earlbaum.

Dijkstra, T., & van Heuven, W. J. B. (2002). The architecture of the bilingual word recognition system: From identification to decision. *Bilingualism: Language and Cognition 5*(3), 175–197.

Dijkstra, T., Van Heuven, W. J. B., & Grainger, J. (1998). Simulating cross-language competition with the bilingual interactive activation model. *Psychologica Belgica, 38*, 177–196.

Dong, Y., & Li, P. (2014). The cognitive science of bilingualism. *Language and Linguistic Compass* (in press).

Dong, Y., & Lin, J. (2013). Parallel processing of the target language during source language comprehension in interpreting. *Bilingualism: Language and Cognition, 16*(3), 682–692.

Eriksen, B. A., & Eriksen, C. W. (1974). Effects of noiseletters uponthe identification of a target letter in a nonsearch task. *Perception & Psychophysics, 16*(1), 143–149.

Feng, X., Bialystok, E., & Diamond, A. (2009). Do Bilingual Children show an Advantage in Working Memory? *1 41.*<http://www.devcogneuro.com/Publications/Feng_Bialystok_Diamond> .

Fernandez, M., Tartar, J. L., Padron, D., & Acosta, J. (2013). Neurophysiological marker of inhibition distinguishes language groups on a non-linguistic executive function test. *Brain and Cognition, 83*(3), 330–336.

Festman, J., & Munte, T. F. (2012). Cognitive control in Russian-german bilinguals. *Frontiers in Psychology, 3*, 115. doi: 10.3389/fpsyg.2012.00115.

Festman, J., Rodriguez-Fornells, A., & Munte, T. F. (2010). Individual differences in control of language interference in late bilinguals are mainly related to general executive abilities. *Behavioral and brain functions, 6*, 5. doi: 10.1186/1744-9081-6-5.

Filippi, R., Karaminis, T., & Thomas, M. S. C. (2013). Language switching in bilingual production: empirical data and computational modelling *Manuscript submitted for publication.*

Fineman, S. (2008). Linking Cognitive Control & Stress Regulation: A Brain-Based Perspective on Self-Regulatory Processes doi: Available electronically from <http://hdl.handle.net/10066/1426>.

Finkbeiner, Gollan, & Caramazza. (2006). Lexical access in bilingual speakers: What's the (hard) problem? *Bilingualism, 9*(02), 153–166.

Finkbeiner, M., Almeida, J., Janssen, N., & Caramazza, A. (2006). Lexical selection in bilingual speech production does not involve language suppression. *Journal of experimental psychology. Learning, memory, and cognition, 32*(5), 1075–1089.

Friedman, N. P., & Miyake, A. (2004). The relations among inhibition and interference control functions: a latent-variable analysis. *Journal of Experimental Psychology: General, 133*(1), 101–135.

Friedman, N. P., Miyake, A., Corley, R. P., Young, S. E., Defries, J. C., & Hewitt, J. K. (2006). Not all executive functions are related to intelligence. *Psychological Science, 17*(2), 172–179.

Gao, L. (2009). Can Executive Skills Help Underachieving Bilingual Students?Pedagogical implications. In M. S. Plakhotnik, S. M. Nielsen, & D. M. Pane (Eds.), . *Proceedings of the Eighth Annual College of Education & GSN Research Conference* (pp. 33–38) Miami: Florida International University <http://coeweb.fiu.edu/research_conference/>.

Garbin, G., Costa, A., Sanjuan, A., Forn, C., Rodriguez-Pujadas, A., Ventura, N., … Avila, C. (2011). Neural bases of language switching in high and early proficient bilinguals. *Brain and Language, 119*(3), 129–135.

Garbin, G., Sanjuan, A., Forn, C., Bustamante, J. C., Rodriguez-Pujadas, A., Belloch, V., … Avila, C. (2010). Bridging language and attention: brain basis of the impact of bilingualism on cognitive control. *Neuroimage, 53*(4), 1272–1278.

Gathercole, V. C., Thomas, E. M., Kennedy, I., Prys, C., Young, N., Vinas Guasch, N., … Jones, L. (2014b). Does language dominance affect cognitive performance in bilinguals? Lifespan evidence from preschoolers through older adults on card sorting, Simon, and metalinguistic tasks. *Frontiers in Psychology, 5*, 11. doi: 10.3389/fpsyg.2014.00011.

Girelli, L., Sandrini, M., Cappa, S., & Butterworth, B. (2001). Number-stroop performance in normal aging and Alzheimer's-type dementia. *Brain and Cognition, 46*(1–2), 144–149.

Gold, B. T., Kim, C., Johnson, N. F., Kryscio, R. J., & Smith, C. D. (2013). Lifelong Bilingualism Maintains Neural Efficiency for Cognitive Control in Aging. *Journal of Neuroscience, 33*(2), 387–396.

Gollan, T. H., & Ferreira, V. S. (2007). *Natural language switching: Expanding the role of inhibitory control*. Paper presented at the the 48th annual meeting of the psychonomic society.

Gollan, T. H., Montoya, R. I., Cera, C., & Sandoval, T. C. (2008). More use almost always means a smaller frequency effect: Aging, bilingualism, and the weaker links hypothesis. *Journal of Memory and Language, 58*(3), 787–814.

Grainger, J., & Dijkstra, A. T. (1992). On the representation and use of language information in bilinguals. In R. J. Harris (Ed.), *Cognitive processing in bilinguals* (pp. 207–220). Amsterdam: Elsevier.

Green, D. W. (1986). Control, activation, and resource: A framework and a model for the control of speech in bilinguals. *Brain and Language, 27*(2), 210–223.

Green, D. W. (1998). Mental control of the bilingual lexico semantic system. *Bilingualism: Language and Cognition, 1*(02), 67–81.

Green, D. W. (2011). Language control in different contexts: the behavioral ecology of bilingual speakers. *Frontiers in Psychology, 2*, 103. doi: 10.3389/fpsyg.2011.00103.

Green, D. W., & Abutalebi, J. (2013). Language control in bilinguals: The adaptive control hypothesis. *Journal of Cognitive Psychology, 25*(5), 515–530.

Greenberg, A., Bellana, B., & Bialystok, E. (2013). Perspective-taking ability in bilingual children: Extending advantages in executive control to spatial reasoning. *Cognitive Development, 28*(1), 41–50.

Grosjean, F. (1985). The bilingual as a competent but specific speaker-hearer. *Journal of Multilingual and Multicultural Development, 6*, 467–477.

Grosjean, F. (1997). Processing mixed language: Issues, findings and models. In A. M. B. DeGroot & J. F. Kroll (Eds.), *Tutorials in Bilingualism: Psycholinguistic Perspectives* (pp. 225–254). Mahwah, NJ: LEA.

Hackman, D. A., & Farah, M. J. (2009). Socioeconomic status and the developing brain. *Trends in Cognitive Sciences, 13*(2), 65–73.

Han, S., & Ma, Y. (2014). Cultural differences in human brain activity: A quantitative meta-analysis. *Neuroimage*. doi: 10.1016/j.neuroimage.2014.05.062.

Harb, G. C., Eng, W., Zaider, T., & Heimberg, R. G. (2003). Behavioral assessment of public-speaking anxiety using a modified version of the Social Performance Rating Scale. *Behaviour Research and Therapy, 41*(11), 1373–1380.

Hartman, M., Bolton, E., & Fehnel, S. E. (2001). Accounting for age difference on the wisconsin card sorting test: decreased working memory, not inflexibility. *Psychology and Aging, 16*(3), 385–399.

Hartman, M., Steketee, M. C., Silva, S., Lanning, K., & Andersson, C. (2003). Wisconsin Card Sorting Test performance in schizophrenia: the role of working memory. *Schizophrenia Research, 63*(3), 201–217.

Heaton, R. K., Chelune, G. L., Talley, J. L., Kay, G. G., Gary, R. J., & Curtiss, G. (1993). *Wisconsin Card Sorting Test Manual – Revised and Expanded*. Odessa: Psychological Assessment Resources.

Hernández, M., Costa, A., Fuentes, L. J., Vivas, A. B., & Sebastián-Gallés, N. (2010). The impact of bilingualism on the executive control and orienting networks of attention. *Bilingualism: Language and Cognition, 13*(03), 315–325.

Hervais-Adelman, A., Moser-Mercer, B., Michel, C. M., & Golestani, N. (2014). fMRI of Simultaneous Interpretation Reveals the Neural Basis of Extreme Language Control. *Cerebral Cortex*. doi: 10.1093/cercor/bhu158.

Hervais-Adelman, A. G., Moser-Mercer, B., & Golestani, N. (2011). Executive control of language in the bilingual brain: integrating the evidence from neuroimaging to neuropsychology. *Frontiers in Psychology, 2*, 234. doi: 10.3389/fpsyg.2011.00234.

Hilchey, M. D., & Klein, R. M. (2011). Are there bilingual advantages on nonlinguistic interference tasks? Implications for the plasticity of executive control processes. *Psychonomic Bulletin and Review, 18*(4), 625–658.

Hommel, B., Colzato, L. S., Fischer, R., & Christoffels, I. K. (2011). Bilingualism and creativity: benefits in convergent thinking come with losses in divergent thinking. *Frontiers in Psychology, 2*, 273. doi: 10.3389/fpsyg.2011.00273.

Hook, Lawson, & Farah. (2013). Socioeconomic Status and the Development of Executive Function *Encyclopedia on Early Childhood Development* 1–7 <http://www.child-encyclopedia.com/documents/Hook- Lawson-FarahANGxp1.pdf>.

Hoshino, N., & Kroll, J. F. (2008). Cognate effects in picture naming: does cross-language activation survive a change of script? *Cognition, 106*(1), 501–511.

Hoshino, N., & Thierry, G. (2011). Language selection in bilingual word production: electrophysiological evidence for cross-language competition. *Brain Research, 1371*, 100–109.

Hulstijn, J. H. (2012). The construct of language proficiency in the study of bilingualism from a cognitive perspective. *Bilingualism: Language and Cognition, 15*(02), 422–433.

Humphrey, A. D., & Valian, V. V. (2012). *Multilingualism and cognitive control:Simon and flanker task performance in monolingual and multilingual young adults*. Paper presented at the 53rd Annual meeting of the psychonomic society, Minneapolis, MN.

Hussey, E. K., & Novick, J. M. (2012). The benefits of executive control training and the implications for language processing. *Frontiers in Psychology, 3*, 158. doi: 10.3389/fpsyg.2012.00158.

Ibanez, A. J., Macizo, P., & Bajo, M. T. (2010). Language access and language selection in professional translators. *Acta Psychologica (Amst), 135*(2), 257–266.
Iluz-Cohen, P., & Armon-Lotem, S. (2013). Language proficiency and executive control in bilingual children. *Bilingualism: Language and Cognition, 16*(04), 884–899.
Jackson, G. M., Swainson, R., Cunnington, R., & Jackson, S. R. (2001). ERP correlates of executive control during repeated language switching. *Bilingualism: Language and Cognition, 4*(02), 169–178.
Jersild, A. T. (1927). Mental set and shift. *Archives Psychol, 89.*
Jones, C. R., Fazio, R. H., & Vasey, M. W. (2012). Attentional Control Buffers the Effect of Public Speaking Anxiety on Performance. *Social psychological and personality science, 3*(5), 556–561.
Kar, B. R., Khare, V., & Dash, T. (2011). Bilingualism and Cognitive control: Is bilingualism a cognitive advantage? . In R. K. Mishra & N. Srinivasan (Eds.), *Language and Cognition: State of the Art*. Munich: Lincom Europa.
Kaushanskaya, M., & Prior, A. (2014). Variability in the effects of bilingualism on cognition: It is not just about cognition, it is also about bilingualism. *Bilingualism: Language and Cognition, 18*(01), 27–28.
Kave, Eyal, Shorek, & Cohen-Mansfield. (2008). Multilingualism and cognitive state in the oldest old. *Psychology and Aging, 23*(1), 70–78.
Kharkhurin, A. V. (2011). The Role of Selective Attention in Bilingual Creativity. *Creativity Research Journal, 23*(3), 239–254.
Khateb, A., Abutalebi, J., Michel, C. M., Pegna, A. J., Lee-Jahnke, H., & Annoni, J. M. (2007). Language selection in bilinguals: a spatio-temporal analysis of electric brain activity. *International Journal of Psychophysiology, 65*(3), 201–213.
Kirk, N. W., Fiala, L., Scott-Brown, K. C., & Kempe, V. (2014). No evidence for reduced Simon cost in elderly bilinguals and bidialectals. *Journal of Cognitive Psychology (Hove), 26*(6), 640–648.
Klimkeit, E. I., Mattingley, J. B., Sheppard, D. M., Farrow, M., & Bradshaw, J. L. (2004). Examining the development of attention and

executive functions in children with a novel paradigm. *Child Neuropsychology, 10*(3), 201–211.

Kormos, J. (2006). *Speech Production and Second Language Acquisition*. New Jersey: Lawrence Erlbaum Associates.

Kousaie, S. (2011). *A behavioural and electrophysiological investigation of the "bilingual advantage"* Doctor of Philosophy, Concordia University.

Kousaie, S., & Phillips, N. A. (2012a). Ageing and bilingualism: absence of a "bilingual advantage" in stroop interference in a nonimmigrant sample. *The Quarterly Journal of Experimental Psychology 65*(2), 356–369.

Kousaie, S., & Phillips, N. A. (2012b). Conflict monitoring and resolution: are two languages better than one? Evidence from reaction time and event-related brain potentials. *Brain Research, 1446*, 71–90.

Kousaie, S., Sheppard, C., Lemieux, M., Monetta, L., & Taler, V. (2014). Executive function and bilingualism in young and older adults. *Frontiers in Behavioral Neuroscience, 8*, 250. doi: 10.3389/fnbeh.2014.00250.

Kroll, J. F., & Bialystok, E. (2013). Understanding the Consequences of Bilingualism for Language Processing and Cognition. *Journal of Cognitive Psychology, 25*(5), 497–514.

Kroll, J. F., Bobb, S. C., Misra, M., & Guo, T. (2008). Language selection in bilingual speech: evidence for inhibitory processes. *Acta Psychologica 128*(3), 416–430.

Kutas, M., & Van Petten, C. K. (1994). Psycholinguistics electrified: Event-related brain potential investigations. In M. A. Gernsbacher (Ed.), *Handbook of psycholinguistics* (pp. 83–143). San Diego, CA: Academic Press, Inc.

LaHeij, W., Vander Heijden, A. H. C., & Schreuder, R. (1985). Semantic priming and Stroop-like interference in word-naming tasks. *Journal of Experimental Psychology: Human Perception and Performance, 11*, 62–80.

Leikin, M. (2012). The effect of bilingualism on creativity: Developmental and educational perspectives. *International Journal of Bilingualism*. 17(4), 431–447.

Leon-Carrion, J., García-Orza, J., & Pérez-Santamaría, F. J. (2004). Development of the inhibitory component of the executive functions in children and adolescents. *International Journal of Neuroscience, 114*(10), 1291–1311.

Levelt, W. J. M. (1989). *Speaking: from intention to articulation*. Cambridge, Massachusetts: The MIT Press.

Linck, J. A., Kroll, J. F., & Sunderman, G. (2009). Losing access to the native language while immersed in a second language: evidence for the role of inhibition in second-language learning. *Psychological Science, 20*(12), 1507–1515.

Linck, J. A., Schwieter, J. W., & Sunderman, G. (2011). Inhibitory control predicts language switching performance in trilingual speech production. *Bilingualism: Language and Cognition, 15*(03), 651–662.

Losel, F., & Schmucker, M. (2004). Psychopathy, risktaking, and attention: A differentiated test of the somatic marker hypothesis. *Journal of Abnormal Psychology, 113*, 522–529.

Lovett, M. C. (2002). Modeling selective attention: Not just another model of Stroop (NJAMOS). . *Cognitive Systems Research, 3*(1), 67–76.

Luciana, M., & Nelson, C. A. (2002). Assessment of neuropsychological function through use of the Cambridge Neuropsychological Testing Automated Battery: Performance in 4- to 12-year old children. *Developmental Neuropsychology, 22*(3), 595–624.

Luk, G., Anderson, J. A., Craik, F. I., Grady, C., & Bialystok, E. (2010). Distinct neural correlates for two types of inhibition in bilinguals: response inhibition versus interference suppression. *Brain and Cognition, 74*(3), 347–357.

Luk, G., & Bialystok, E. (2013). Bilingualism is not a categorical variable: Interaction between language proficiency and usage. *Journal of Cognitive Psychology, 25*(5), 605–621.

Luk, G., Green, D. W., Abutalebi, J., & Grady, C. (2012). Cognitive control for language switching in bilinguals: A quantitative meta-analysis of functional neuroimaging studies. *Language and Cognitive Processes, 27*(10), 1479–1488.

Luna, B., Garver, K. E., Urban, T. A., Lazar, N. A., & Sweeney, J. A. (2004). Maturation of cognitive processes from late childhood to adulthood. *Child Development Research, 75*(5), 1357–1372.

Luo, L., Luk, G., & Bialystok, E. (2010). Effect of language proficiency and executive control on verbal fluency performance in bilinguals. *Cognition, 114*(1), 29–41.

Lupker, S. J. (1979). The semantic nature of response competition in the picture-word interference task. *Memory and Cognition, 7*, 485–495.

Lupker, S. J. (1982). The role of phonetic and orthographic similarity in picture-word interference. *Canadian Journal of Psychology, 36*, 349–367.

Macnamara, B. N., & Conway, A. R. (2014). Novel evidence in support of the bilingual advantage: influences of task demands and experience on cognitive control and working memory. *Psychonomic Bulletin and Review, 21*(2), 520–525.

Macnamara, J., & Kushnir, S. L. (1971). Linguistic independence of bilinguals: The input switch. *Journal of Verbal Learning and Verbal Behavior, 10*(5), 480–487.

Magezi, D. A., Khateb, A., Mouthon, M., Spierer, L., & Annoni, J. M. (2012). Cognitive control of language production in bilinguals involves a partly independent process within the domain-general cognitive control network: evidence from task-switching and electrical brain activity. *Brain and Language, 122*(1), 55–63.

Marian, V., Blumenfeld, H. K., & Kaushanskaya, M. (2007). The Language Experience and Proficiency Questionnaire(LEAP-Q): Assessing Language Profiles in Bilinguals and Multilinguals. *Journal of Speech,Language,and Hearing Research, 50*, 940–967.

Marian, V., Blumenfeld, H. K., Mizrahi, E., Kania, U., & Cordes, A. K. (2013). Multilingual Stroop performance: Effects of trilingualism and proficiency on inhibitory control. *International Journal of Multilingualism, 10*(1), 82–104.

Martin-Rhee, M. M., & Bialystok, E. (2008). The development of two types of inhibitory control in monolingual and bilingual children. *Bilingualism: Language and Cognition, 11*(01), 81–93.

Marzecová, A., Bukowski, M., Correa, Á., Boros, M., Lupiáñez, J., & Wodniecka, Z. (2013). Tracing the bilingual advantage in cognitive control: The role of flexibility in temporal preparation and category switching. *Journal of Cognitive Psychology, 25*(5), 586–604.

Meuter, R. F. I., & Allport, A. (1999). Bilingual Language Switching in Naming: Asymmetrical Costs of Language Selection. *Journal of Memory and Language, 40*, 25–40.

Miller, & Cohen. (2001). AN INTEGRATIVE THEORYOF PREFRONTAL CORTEX FUNCTION. *Annu.Rev.Neurosci., 24*, 167–202.

Millner, A. J., Jaroszewski, A. C., Chamarthi, H., & Pizzagalli, D. A. (2012). Behavioral and electrophysiological correlates of training-induced cognitive control improvements. *Neuroimage, 63*(2), 742–753.

Mishra, R. K., Hilchey, M. D., Singh, N., & Klein, R. M. (2012). On the time course of exogenous cueing effects in bilinguals: higher proficiency in a second language is associated with more rapid endogenous disengagement. *Quarterly Journal of Experimental Psychology, 65*(8), 1502–1510.

Miyake, A., & Friedman, N. P. (2012). The Nature and Organization of Individual Differences in Executive Functions: Four General Conclusions. *Current Directions in Psychological Science, 21*(1), 8–14.

Miyake, A., Friedman, N. P., Emerson, M. J., Witzki, A. H., Howerter, A., & Wager, T. D. (2000). The unity and diversity of executive functions and their contributions to complex "Frontal Lobe" tasks: a latent variable analysis. *Cognitive Psychology, 41*(1), 49–100.

Monsell, S. (1996). Control of mental processes. In V. Bruce (Ed.), *Unsolved mysteries of the mind: Tutorial essays in cognition.* Hove, U.K.: Erlbaum, Taylor & Francis.

Monsell, S. (2003). Task switching. *Trends in Cognitive Sciences, 7*(3), 134–140.

Morales, J., Calvo, A., & Bialystok, E. (2013). Working memory development in monolingual and bilingual children. *J Exp Child Psychol, 114*(2), 187–202.

Morales, J., Padilla, F., Gomez-Ariza, C. J., & Bajo, M. T. (2015). Simultaneous interpretation selectively influences working memory and attentional networks. *Acta Psychologica (Amst), 155C*, 82–91.

Morales, J., Yudes, C., Gomez-Ariza, C. J., & Bajo, M. T. (2015). Bilingualism modulates dual mechanisms of cognitive control: Evidence from ERPs. *Neuropsychologia, 66*, 157–169.

Moreno, E. M., Rodrıguez-Fornells, A., & Laine, M. (2008). Event-related potentials (ERPs) in the study of bilingual language processing. *Journal of Neurolinguistics, 21*(6), 477–508.

Moreno, S., Wodniecka, Z., Tays, W., Alain, C., & Bialystok, E. (2014). Inhibitory control in bilinguals and musicians: event related potential (ERP) evidence for experience-specific effects. *PLoS One, 9*(4), e94169. doi: 10.1371/journal.pone.0094169.

Mueller, S. C. (2011). The influence of emotion on cognitive control: relevance for development and adolescent psychopathology. *Frontiers in Psychology, 2*, 327. doi: 10.3389/fpsyg.2011.00327.

Noble, K. G., Norman, M. F., & Farah, M. J. (2005). Neurocognitive correlates of socioeconomic status in kindergarten children. *Developmental Science, 8*(1), 74–87.

Norman, D. A., & Shallice, T. (1980). Attention to action: Willed and automatic control of behaviour. Reprinted In M. Gazzaniga (Ed.), *(2000) Cognitive Neuroscience: A Reader*: Blackwell.

Nyhus, E., & Barcelo, F. (2009). The Wisconsin Card Sorting Test and the cognitive assessment of prefrontal executive functions: a critical update. *Brain and Cognition, 71*(3), 437–451.

Paap, K. R. (2014). The role of componential analysis, categorical hypothesising, replicability and confirmation bias in testing for bilingual advantages in executive functioning. *Journal of Cognitive Psychology, 26*(3), 242–255.

Paap, K. R., & Greenberg, Z. I. (2013). There is no coherent evidence for a bilingual advantage in executive processing. *Cognitive Psychology, 66*(2), 232–258.

Padilla, F., Bajo, M. T., & Macizo, P. (2005). Articulatory suppression in language interpretation: Working memory capacity, dual tasking and word knowledge. *Bilingualism: Language and Cognition, 8*(03), 207–219.

Paradis, M. (1981). Neurolinguistic organization of a bilingual's twol anguages. In J. E. Copeland & P. W. Davis (Eds.), *The seventh LACUS Forum* (pp. 486–494). Columbia, SC: Hornbeam Press.

Paradis, M. (2004). *A neurolinguistic theory of bilingualism*. Amsterdam: John Benjamins.

Parker, J., Green, D. W., Grogan, A., Pliatsikas, C., Filippopolitis, K., Ali, N., … Price, C. J. (2012). Where, when and why brain activation differs for bilinguals and monolinguals during picture naming and reading aloud. *Cerebral Cortex, 22*(4), 892–902.

Paulmann, S., Elston-Guttler, K. E., Gunter, T. C., & Kotz, S. A. (2006). Is bilingual lexical access influenced by language context? *NeuroReport, 17*(7), 727–731.

Peal, E., & Lambert, W. E. (1962). The Relation Of Bilingualism To Intelligence. *Psychological Monographs: General and Applied 76*, 1–23.

Pearson, B. Z., Fernandez, S. C., & Oller, D. K. (1993). Lexical development in bilingual infants andbtoddlers: Comparison to monolingual norms. *Language Learning, 43*(1), 93–120.

Penfield, W., & Roberts, L. (1959). *Speech and Brain Mechanisms*. Princeton, NJ: Princeton University Press.

Pivneva, I., Palmer, C., & Titone, D. (2012). Inhibitory control and L2 proficiency modulate bilingual language production: evidence from spontaneous monologue and dialogue speech. *Frontiers in Psychology, 3*, 57. doi: 10.3389/fpsyg.2012.00057.

Poulisse, N. (1997). Language production in bilinguals. In A. M. B. de Groot & F. J. Kroll (Eds.), *Tutorials in bilingualism: Psycholinguistic perspectives* (pp. 201–224). Mahwah, NJ: Erlbaum.

Pribyl, C. B., Keaten, J., & Sakamoto, M. (2001). The effectiveness of a skills-based program in reducing public speaking anxiety. *Japanese Psychological Research, 43*(3), 148–155.

Prior, A., & Gollan, T. H. (2011). Good language-switchers are good task-switchers: evidence from Spanish-English and Mandarin-English bilinguals. *Journal of the International Neuropsychological Society, 17*(4), 682–691.

Prior, A., & Macwhinney, B. (2010). A bilingual advantage in task switching. *Bilingualism: Language and Cognition, 13*(02), 253–262.

Proverbio, A. M., Čok, B., & Zani, A. (2002). Electrophysiological measures of language processing in bilinguals. *Journal of Cognitive Neuroscience, 14*(7), 994–1017.

Pyers, J. E., Gollan, T. H., & Emmorey, K. (2009). Bimodal bilinguals reveal the source of tip-of-the-tongue states. *Cognition, 112*(2), 323–329.

Raven, J. C., Court, J. H., & Raven, J. (1977). *Manual for Raven's advanced progressive matrices:Sets I and II.* London,England: H.K. Lewis&Co.Ltd.

Ricciardelli, L. A. (1992). Creativity and Bilingualism. *The Journal of Creative Behavior, 26*(4), 242–254.

Rodriguez-Fornells, A., Balaguer, R. D. D., & Munte, T. F. (2006). Executive Control in Bilingual Language Processing. *Language Learning, 56*, 133–190.

Rodriguez-Fornells, A., Kramer, U. M., Lorenzo-Seva, U., Festman, J., & Munte, T. F. (2011). Self-assessment of individual differences in language switching. *Frontiers in Psychology, 2*, 388. doi: 10.3389/fpsyg.2011.00388.

Rodriguez-Fornells, A., Lugt, A., Rotte, M., BelindanBritti, Heinze, H.-J., & F.Munte, T. (2005). Second Language Interferes with Word Production in Fluent Bilinguals:Brain Potential and Functional Imaging Evidence. *Journal of Cognitive Neuroscience, 17*(3), 422–433.

Rodriguez-Fornells, A., Rotte, M., Heinze, H. J., Nosselt, T., & Munte, T. F. (2002). Brain potential and functional MRI evidence for how to handle two languages with one brain. *Nature, 415*(6875), 1026–1029.

Rodriguez-Pujadas, A., Sanjuan, A., Fuentes, P., Ventura-Campos, N., Barros-Loscertales, A., & Avila, C. (2014). Differential neural control in early bilinguals and monolinguals during response inhibition. *Brain and Language, 132C*, 43–51.

Roelofs, A. (1998). Lemma selection without inhibition of languages in bilingual speakers. *Bilingualism: Language and Cognition, 1*, 94–95.

Rosenblum, T., & Pinker, S. A. (1983). Word magic revisited: Monolingual and bilingual children's understanding of the word-object relationship. *Child Development, 54*, 773–780.

Rosenzweig, M. R. (2003). Effects of differential experience on the brain and behavior. *DevelopmentalNeuropsychology, 24*(2–3), 523–540.

Rubio-Fernández, & Glucksberg. (2012). Reasoning about other people's beliefs: Bilinguals have an advantage. *Journal of Experimental Psychology: Learning, Memory, and Cognition, 38*(1), 211–217.

Runnqvist, E., Strijkers, K., Sadat, J., & Costa, A. (2011). On the temporal and functional origin of l2 disadvantages in speech production: a critical review. *Frontiers in Psychology, 2*, 379. doi: 10.3389/fpsyg.2011.00379.

Saer, D. J. (1923). The Effect of Bilingualism on Intelligence. *British Journal of Psychology: General Section, 14*(1), 25–38.

Salvatierra, J. L., & Rosselli, M. (2011). The effect of bilingualism and age on inhibitory control. *International Journal of Bilingualism, 15*(1), 26–37.

Schel, M. A., & Crone, E. A. (2013). Development of response inhibition in the context of relevant versus irrelevant emotions. *Frontiers in Psychology, 4*, 383. doi: 10.3389/fpsyg.2013.00383.

Schwartz, A. I., Kroll, J. F., & Diaz, M. (2007). Reading words in Spanish and English: Mapping orthography to phonology in two languages. *Language and Cognitive Processes, 22*(1), 106–129.

Schweizer, Ware, Fischer, Craik, & Bialystok. (2012). Bilingualism as a contributor to cognitive reserve: Evidence from brain atrophy in Alzheimer's disease. *Cortex, 48*, 991–996.

Schweizer, T. A., Craik, F. I. M., & Bialystok, E. (2013). Bilingualism, not immigration status, is associated with maintained cognitive level in Alzheimer's disease. *Cortex, 49*(5), 1442–1443.

Senn, T. E., Espy, K. A., & Kaufmann, P. M. (2004). Using path analysis to understand executive function organization in preschool children. *Developmental Neuropsychology, 26*(1), 445–464.

Shao, Z., Roelofs, A., Acheson, D. J., & Meyer, A. S. (2014). Electrophysiological evidence that inhibition supports lexical selection in picture naming. *Brain Research, 1586*, 130–142.

Simon, J. R. (1969). Reactions toward the source of stimulation. *Journal of Experimental Psychology, 81*(1), 174–176.

Singh, N., & Mishra, R. K. (2012). Does language proficiency modulate oculomotor control? Evidence from Hindi–English bilinguals. *Bilingualism: Language and Cognition, 15*(04), 771–781.

Singh, N., & Mishra, R. K. (2013). Second language proficiency modulates conflict-monitoring in an oculomotor Stroop task: evidence from Hindi-English bilinguals. *Frontiers in Psychology, 4*, 322. doi: 10.3389/fpsyg.2013.00322.

Smith, F. (1923). Bilingualism and Mental Development. *British Journal of Psychology: General Section, 13*(3), 271–282.

Soliman, A. M. (2014). Bilingual advantages of working memory revisited: A latent variable examination. *Learning and Individual Differences, 32*, 168–177.

Soveri, A., Rodriguez-Fornells, A., & Laine, M. (2011). Is There a Relationship between Language Switching and Executive Functions in Bilingualism? Introducing a within group Analysis Approach. *Frontiers in Psychology, 2*, 183. doi: 10.3389/fpsyg.2011.00183.

Spreen, O., & Strauss, E. H. (1998). *A Compendium of neuropsychological tests: Administration, norms, and commentary. (2nd ed.).* NY: Oxford University Press.

Stocco, A., Yamasaki, B., Natalenko, R., & Prat, C. S. (2012). Bilingual brain training: A neurobiological framework of how bilingual experience improves executive function. *International Journal of Bilingualism, 18*(1), 67–92.

Stroop, J. R. (1935). Studies of interference in serial verbal reactions *Journal of Experimental Psychology, 18*, 643–662.

Sullivan, M. D., Janus, M., Moreno, S., Astheimer, L., & Bialystok, E. (2014). Early stage second-language learning improves executive control: Evidence from ERP. *Brain and Language, 139*, 84–98.

Taler, V., Johns, B. T., Young, K., Sheppard, C., & Jones, M. N. (2013). A computational analysis of semantic structure in bilingual verbal fluency performance. *Journal of Memory and Language, 69*, 607–618.

Tao, L., Marzecova, A., Taft, M., Asanowicz, D., & Wodniecka, Z. (2011). The efficiency of attentional networks in early and late bilinguals: the role of age of acquisition. *Frontiers in Psychology, 2*, 123. doi: 10.3389/fpsyg.2011.00123.

Toplak, M. E., Sorge, G. B., Benoit, A., West, R. F., & Stanovich, K. E. (2010). Decision-making and cognitive abilities: A review of associations between Iowa Gambling Task performance, executive functions, and intelligence. *Clinical Psychology Review, 30*(5), 562–581.

Tse, C.-S., & Altarriba, J. (2012). The effects of first- and second-language proficiency on conflict resolution and goal maintenance in bilinguals: Evidence from reaction time distributional analyses in a Stroop task. *Bilingualism: Language and Cognition, 15*(03), 663–676.

Tzelgov, J., Meyer, J., & Henik, A. (1992). Automatic and intentional processing of numerical information. *Journal of Experimental Psychology: Learning, Memory, and Cognition, 18*(1), 166–179.

Tzou, Y. Z., Eslami, Z. R., Chen, H. C., & Vaid, J. (2011). Effect of language proficiency and degree of formal training in simultaneous interpreting on working memory and interpreting performance: Evidence from Mandarin-English speakers. *International Journal of Bilingualism, 16*(2), 213–227.

Valian, V. (2014). Bilingualism and cognition. *Bilingualism: Language and Cognition, 18*(01), 3–24.

van Heuven, W. J., Conklin, K., Coderre, E. L., Guo, T., & Dijkstra, T. (2011). The Influence of Cross-Language Similarity on within- and between-Language Stroop Effects in Trilinguals. *Frontiers in Psychology, 2*, 374. doi: 10.3389/fpsyg.2011.00374.

van Heuven, W. J. B., & Dijkstra, T. (2010). Language comprehension in the bilingual brain: fMRI and ERP support for psycholinguistic models. *Brain Research Reviews, 64*(1), 104–122.

Videsott, G., Della Rosa, P. A., Wiater, W., Franceschini, R., & Abutalebi, J. (2012). How does linguistic competence enhance cognitive functions in children? A study in multilingual children with different linguistic competences. *Bilingualism: Language and Cognition, 15*(04), 884–895.

Wallach, H. S., Safir, M. P., & Bar-Zvi, M. (2009). Virtual reality cognitive behavior therapy for public speaking anxiety: a randomized clinical trial. *Behavior Modification, 33*(3), 314–338.

Weldon, R. B., Mushlin, H., Kim, B., & Sohn, M. H. (2013). The effect of working memory capacity on conflict monitoring. *Acta Psychologica (Amst), 142*(1), 6–14.
West, R. (2003). Neural correlates of cognitive control and conflict detection in the Stroop and digit-location tasks. *Neuropsychologia, 41*(8), 1122–1235.
West, R., Jakubek, K., Wymbs, N., Perry, M., & Moore, K. (2005). Neural correlates of conflict processing. *Experimental Brain Research, 167*(1), 38–48.
Woumans, E., Ceuleers, E., Linden, L. V. d., Szmalec, A., & W., W. D. (2015). Verbal and non-verbal cognitive control in bilinguals and interpreters. *Experimental Psychology: learning, memory and cognition, in press.*
Yudes, C., Macizo, P., & Bajo, T. (2011). The influence of expertise in simultaneous interpreting on non-verbal executive processes. *Frontiers in Psychology, 2*, 309. doi: 10.3389/fpsyg.2011.00309.
Yudes, C., Macizo, P., & Bajo, T. (2012). Coordinating comprehension and production in simultaneous interpreters: Evidence from the Articulatory Suppression Effect. *Bilingualism: Language and Cognition, 15*(02), 329–339.
Yudes, C., Macizo, P., Morales, L., & Bajo, M. T. (2012). Comprehension and error monitoring in simultaneous interpreters. *Appllied Psycholinguistics, 34*(05), 1039–1057.
Zelazo, Carter, Reznick, & Frye. (1997). Early development of executive function: A problem-solving framework. *Review of General Psychology, 1*(2), 198–226.
Zied, K. M., Philippe, A., Pinon, K., Havet-Thomassin, V., Ghislaine, A., Roy, A., & Le Gall, D. (2004). Bilingualism and adult differences in inhibitory mechanisms: Evidence from a bilingual Stroop task. *Brain and Cognition, 54*, 254–256.

Linguistic Insights

Studies in Language and Communication

This series aims to promote specialist language studies in the fields of linguistic theory and applied linguistics, by publishing volumes that focus on specific aspects of language use in one or several languages and provide valuable insights into language and communication research. A cross-disciplinary approach is favoured and most European languages are accepted.

The series includes two types of books:

- **Monographs** – featuring in-depth studies on special aspects of language theory, language analysis or language teaching.
- **Collected papers** – assembling papers from workshops, conferences or symposia.

Each volume of the series is subjected to a double peer-reviewing process.

Vol. 1 Maurizio Gotti & Marina Dossena (eds)
Modality in Specialized Texts. Selected Papers of the 1st CERLIS Conference.
421 pages. 2001. ISBN 3-906767-10-8 · US-ISBN 0-8204-5340-4

Vol. 2 Giuseppina Cortese & Philip Riley (eds)
Domain-specific English. Textual Practices across Communities and Classrooms.
420 pages. 2002. ISBN 3-906768-98-8 · US-ISBN 0-8204-5884-8

Vol. 3 Maurizio Gotti, Dorothee Heller & Marina Dossena (eds)
Conflict and Negotiation in Specialized Texts. Selected Papers of the 2nd CERLIS Conference.
470 pages. 2002. ISBN 3-906769-12-7 · US-ISBN 0-8204-5887-2

Vol. 4 Maurizio Gotti, Marina Dossena, Richard Dury, Roberta Facchinetti & Maria Lima
Variation in Central Modals. A Repertoire of Forms and Types of Usage in Middle English and Early Modern English.
364 pages. 2002. ISBN 3-906769-84-4 · US-ISBN 0-8204-5898-8

Editorial address:

Prof. Maurizio Gotti Università di Bergamo, Dipartimento di Lingue, Letterature Straniere e Comunicazione, Piazza Rosate 2, 24129 Bergamo, Italy
Fax: +39 035 2052789, E-Mail: m.gotti@unibg.it

Vol. 5 Stefania Nuccorini (ed.)
Phrases and Phraseology. Data and Descriptions.
187 pages. 2002. ISBN 3-906770-08-7 · US-ISBN 0-8204-5933-X

Vol. 6 Vijay Bhatia, Christopher N. Candlin & Maurizio Gotti (eds)
Legal Discourse in Multilingual and Multicultural Contexts.
Arbitration Texts in Europe.
385 pages. 2003. ISBN 3-906770-85-0 · US-ISBN 0-8204-6254-3

Vol. 7 Marina Dossena & Charles Jones (eds)
Insights into Late Modern English. 2nd edition.
378 pages. 2003, 2007.
ISBN 978-3-03911-257-9 · US-ISBN 978-0-8204-8927-8

Vol. 8 Maurizio Gotti
Specialized Discourse. Linguistic Features and Changing Conventions.
351 pages. 2003, 2005.
ISBN 3-03910-606-6 · US-ISBN 0-8204-7000-7

Vol. 9 Alan Partington, John Morley & Louann Haarman (eds)
Corpora and Discourse.
420 pages. 2004. ISBN 3-03910-026-2 · US-ISBN 0-8204-6262-4

Vol. 10 Martina Möllering
The Acquisition of German Modal Particles. A Corpus-Based Approach.
290 pages. 2004. ISBN 3-03910-043-2 · US-ISBN 0-8204-6273-X

Vol. 11 David Hart (ed.)
English Modality in Context. Diachronic Perspectives.
261 pages. 2003. ISBN 3-03910-046-7 · US-ISBN 0-8204-6852-5

Vol. 12 Wendy Swanson
Modes of Co-reference as an Indicator of Genre.
430 pages. 2003. ISBN 3-03910-052-1 · US-ISBN 0-8204-6855-X

Vol. 13 Gina Poncini
Discursive Strategies in Multicultural Business Meetings.
2nd edition. 338 pages. 2004, 2007.
ISBN 978-3-03911-296-8 · US-ISBN 978-0-8204-8937-7

Vol. 14 Christopher N. Candlin & Maurizio Gotti (eds)
Intercultural Aspects of Specialized Communication.
2nd edition. 369 pages. 2004, 2007.
ISBN 978-3-03911-258-6 · US-ISBN 978-0-8204-8926-1

Vol. 15 Gabriella Del Lungo Camiciotti & Elena Tognini Bonelli (eds)
Academic Discourse. New Insights into Evaluation.
234 pages. 2004. ISBN 3-03910-353-9 · US-ISBN 0-8204-7016-3

Vol. 16 Marina Dossena & Roger Lass (eds)
Methods and Data in English Historical Dialectology.
405 pages. 2004. ISBN 3-03910-362-8 · US-ISBN 0-8204-7018-X

Vol. 17 Judy Noguchi
The Science Review Article. An Opportune Genre in
the Construction of Science.
274 pages. 2006. ISBN 3-03910-426-8 · US-ISBN 0-8204-7034-1

Vol. 18 Giuseppina Cortese & Anna Duszak (eds)
Identity, Community, Discourse. English in Intercultural Settings.
495 pages. 2005. ISBN 3-03910-632-5 · US-ISBN 0-8204-7163-1

Vol. 19 Anna Trosborg & Poul Erik Flyvholm Jørgensen (eds)
Business Discourse. Texts and Contexts.
250 pages. 2005. ISBN 3-03910-606-6 · US-ISBN 0-8204-7000-7

Vol. 20 Christopher Williams
Tradition and Change in Legal English. Verbal Constructions in Prescriptive Texts.
2nd revised edition. 216 pages. 2005, 2007. ISBN 978-3-03911-444-3.

Vol. 21 Katarzyna Dziubalska-Kolaczyk & Joanna Przedlacka (eds)
English Pronunciation Models: A Changing Scene.
2nd edition. 476 pages. 2005, 2008. ISBN 978-3-03911-682-9.

Vol. 22 Christián Abello-Contesse, Rubén Chacón-Beltrán, M. Dolores López-Jiménez & M. Mar Torreblanca-López (eds)
Age in L2 Acquisition and Teaching.
214 pages. 2006. ISBN 3-03910-668-6 · US-ISBN 0-8204-7174-7

Vol. 23 Vijay K. Bhatia, Maurizio Gotti, Jan Engberg & Dorothee Heller (eds)
Vagueness in Normative Texts.
474 pages. 2005. ISBN 3-03910-653-8 · US-ISBN 0-8204-7169-0

Vol. 24 Paul Gillaerts & Maurizio Gotti (eds)
Genre Variation in Business Letters. 2nd printing.
407 pages. 2008. ISBN 978-3-03911-681-2.

Vol. 25 Ana María Hornero, María José Luzón & Silvia Murillo (eds)
Corpus Linguistics. Applications for the Study of English.
2nd printing. 526 pages. 2006, 2008. ISBN 978-3-03911-726-0

Vol. 26 J. Lachlan Mackenzie & María de los Ángeles Gómez-González (eds)
Studies in Functional Discourse Grammar.
259 pages. 2005. ISBN 3-03910-696-1 · US-ISBN 0-8204-7558-0

Vol. 27 Debbie G. E. Ho
Classroom Talk. Exploring the Sociocultural Structure of Formal ESL Learning.
2nd edition. 254 pages. 2006, 2007. ISBN 978-3-03911-434-4

Vol. 28 Javier Pérez-Guerra, Dolores González-Álvarez, Jorge L. Bueno-Alonso & Esperanza Rama-Martínez (eds)
'Of Varying Language and Opposing Creed'. New Insights into Late Modern English.
455 pages. 2007. ISBN 978-3-03910-788-9

Vol. 29 Francesca Bargiela-Chiappini & Maurizio Gotti (eds)
Asian Business Discourse(s).
350 pages. 2005. ISBN 3-03910-804-2 · US-ISBN 0-8204-7574-2

Vol. 30 Nicholas Brownlees (ed.)
News Discourse in Early Modern Britain. Selected Papers of CHINED 2004.
300 pages. 2006. ISBN 3-03910-805-0 · US-ISBN 0-8204-8025-8

Vol. 31 Roberta Facchinetti & Matti Rissanen (eds)
Corpus-based Studies of Diachronic English.
300 pages. 2006. ISBN 3-03910-851-4 · US-ISBN 0-8204-8040-1

Vol. 32 Marina Dossena & Susan M. Fitzmaurice (eds)
Business and Official Correspondence. Historical Investigations.
209 pages. 2006. ISBN 3-03910-880-8 · US-ISBN 0-8204-8352-4

Vol. 33 Giuliana Garzone & Srikant Sarangi (eds)
Discourse, Ideology and Specialized Communication.
494 pages. 2007. ISBN 978-3-03910-888-6

Vol. 34 Giuliana Garzone & Cornelia Ilie (eds)
The Use of English in Institutional and Business Settings.
An Intercultural Perspective.
372 pages. 2007. ISBN 978-3-03910-889-3

Vol. 35 Vijay K. Bhatia & Maurizio Gotti (eds)
Explorations in Specialized Genres.
316 pages. 2006. ISBN 3-03910-995-2 · US-ISBN 0-8204-8372-9

Vol. 36 Heribert Picht (ed.)
Modern Approaches to Terminological Theories and Applications.
432 pages. 2006. ISBN 3-03911-156-6 · US-ISBN 0-8204-8380-X

Vol. 37 Anne Wagner & Sophie Cacciaguidi-Fahy (eds)
Legal Language and the Search for Clarity / Le langage juridique et la quête de clarté.
Practice and Tools / Pratiques et instruments.
487 pages. 2006. ISBN 3-03911-169-8 · US-ISBN 0-8204-8388-5

Vol. 38 Juan Carlos Palmer-Silveira, Miguel F. Ruiz-Garrido &
Inmaculada Fortanet-Gómez (eds)
Intercultural and International Business Communication.
Theory, Research and Teaching.
2nd edition. 343 pages. 2006, 2008. ISBN 978-3-03911-680-5

Vol. 39 Christiane Dalton-Puffer, Dieter Kastovsky, Nikolaus Ritt &
Herbert Schendl (eds)
Syntax, Style and Grammatical Norms. English from 1500–2000.
250 pages. 2006. ISBN 3-03911-181-7 · US-ISBN 0-8204-8394-X

Vol. 40 Marina Dossena & Irma Taavitsainen (eds)
Diachronic Perspectives on Domain-Specific English.
280 pages. 2006. ISBN 3-03910-176-0 · US-ISBN 0-8204-8391-5

Vol. 41 John Flowerdew & Maurizio Gotti (eds)
Studies in Specialized Discourse.
293 pages. 2006. ISBN 3-03911-178-7

Vol. 42 Ken Hyland & Marina Bondi (eds)
Academic Discourse Across Disciplines.
320 pages. 2006. ISBN 3-03911-183-3 · US-ISBN 0-8204-8396-6

Vol. 43 Paul Gillaerts & Philip Shaw (eds)
The Map and the Landscape. Norms and Practices in Genre.
256 pages. 2006. ISBN 3-03911-182-5 · US-ISBN 0-8204-8395-4

Vol. 44 Maurizio Gotti & Davide Giannoni (eds)
New Trends in Specialized Discourse Analysis.
301 pages. 2006. ISBN 3-03911-184-1 · US-ISBN 0-8204-8381-8

Vol. 45 Maurizio Gotti & Françoise Salager-Meyer (eds)
Advances in Medical Discourse Analysis. Oral and Written Contexts.
492 pages. 2006. ISBN 3-03911-185-X · US-ISBN 0-8204-8382-6

Vol. 46 Maurizio Gotti & Susan Šarcević (eds)
Insights into Specialized Translation.
396 pages. 2006. ISBN 3-03911-186-8 · US-ISBN 0-8204-8383-4

Vol. 47 Khurshid Ahmad & Margaret Rogers (eds)
Evidence-based LSP. Translation, Text and Terminology.
584 pages. 2007. ISBN 978-3-03911-187-9

Vol. 48 Hao Sun & Dániel Z. Kádár (eds)
It's the Dragon's Turn. Chinese Institutional Discourses.
262 pages. 2008. ISBN 978-3-03911-175-6

Vol. 49 Cristina Suárez-Gómez
Relativization in Early English (950-1250). the Position of Relative Clauses.
149 pages. 2006. ISBN 3-03911-203-1 · US-ISBN 0-8204-8904-2

Vol. 50 Maria Vittoria Calvi & Luisa Chierichetti (eds)
Nuevas tendencias en el discurso de especialidad.
319 pages. 2006. ISBN 978-3-03911-261-6

Vol. 51 Mari Carmen Campoy & María José Luzón (eds)
Spoken Corpora in Applied Linguistics.
274 pages. 2008. ISBN 978-3-03911-275-3

Vol. 52 Konrad Ehlich & Dorothee Heller (Hrsg.)
Die Wissenschaft und ihre Sprachen.
323 pages. 2006. ISBN 978-3-03911-272-2

Vol. 53 Jingyu Zhang
The Semantic Salience Hierarchy Model. The L2 Acquisition of Psych Predicates
273 pages. 2007. ISBN 978-3-03911-300-2

Vol. 54 Norman Fairclough, Giuseppina Cortese & Patrizia Ardizzone (eds)
Discourse and Contemporary Social Change.
555 pages. 2007. ISBN 978-3-03911-276-0

Vol. 55 Jan Engberg, Marianne Grove Ditlevsen, Peter Kastberg & Martin Stegu (eds)
New Directions in LSP Teaching.
331 pages. 2007. ISBN 978-3-03911-433-7

Vol. 56 Dorothee Heller & Konrad Ehlich (Hrsg.)
Studien zur Rechtskommunikation.
322 pages. 2007. ISBN 978-3-03911-436-8

Vol. 57 Teruhiro Ishiguro & Kang-kwong Luke (eds)
Grammar in Cross-Linguistic Perspective.
The Syntax, Semantics, and Pragmatics of Japanese and Chinese.
304 pages. 2012. ISBN 978-3-03911-445-0

Vol. 58 Carmen Frehner
Email – SMS – MMS
294 pages. 2008. ISBN 978-3-03911-451-1

Vol. 59 Isabel Balteiro
The Directionality of Conversion in English. A Dia-Synchronic Study.
276 pages. 2007. ISBN 978-3-03911-241-8

Vol. 60 Maria Milagros Del Saz Rubio
English Discourse Markers of Reformulation.
237 pages. 2007. ISBN 978-3-03911-196-1

Vol. 61 Sally Burgess & Pedro Martín-Martín (eds)
English as an Additional Language in Research Publication and Communication.
259 pages. 2008. ISBN 978-3-03911-462-7

Vol. 62 Sandrine Onillon
Pratiques et représentations de l'écrit.
458 pages. 2008. ISBN 978-3-03911-464-1

Vol. 63 Hugo Bowles & Paul Seedhouse (eds)
Conversation Analysis and Language for Specific Purposes.
2nd edition. 337 pages. 2007, 2009. ISBN 978-3-0343-0045-2

Vol. 64 Vijay K. Bhatia, Christopher N. Candlin & Paola Evangelisti Allori (eds)
Language, Culture and the Law.
The Formulation of Legal Concepts across Systems and Cultures.
342 pages. 2008. ISBN 978-3-03911-470-2

Vol. 65 Jonathan Culpeper & Dániel Z. Kádár (eds)
Historical (Im)politeness.
300 pages. 2010. ISBN 978-3-03911-496-2

Vol. 66 Linda Lombardo (ed.)
Using Corpora to Learn about Language and Discourse.
237 pages. 2009. ISBN 978-3-03911-522-8

Vol. 67 Natsumi Wakamoto
Extroversion/Introversion in Foreign Language Learning.
Interactions with Learner Strategy Use.
159 pages. 2009. ISBN 978-3-03911-596-9

Vol. 68 Eva Alcón-Soler (ed.)
Learning How to Request in an Instructed Language Learning Context.
260 pages. 2008. ISBN 978-3-03911-601-0

Vol. 69 Domenico Pezzini
The Translation of Religious Texts in the Middle Ages.
428 pages. 2008. ISBN 978-3-03911-600-3

Vol. 70 Tomoko Tode
Effects of Frequency in Classroom Second Language Learning.
Quasi-experiment and stimulated-recall analysis.
195 pages. 2008. ISBN 978-3-03911-602-7

Vol. 71 Egor Tsedryk
Fusion symétrique et alternances ditransitives.
211 pages. 2009. ISBN 978-3-03911-609-6

Vol. 72 Cynthia J. Kellett Bidoli & Elana Ochse (eds)
English in International Deaf Communication.
444 pages. 2008. ISBN 978-3-03911-610-2

Vol. 73 Joan C. Beal, Carmela Nocera & Massimo Sturiale (eds)
Perspectives on Prescriptivism.
269 pages. 2008. ISBN 978-3-03911-632-4

Vol. 74 Carol Taylor Torsello, Katherine Ackerley & Erik Castello (eds)
Corpora for University Language Teachers.
308 pages. 2008. ISBN 978-3-03911-639-3

Vol. 75 María Luisa Pérez Cañado (ed.)
English Language Teaching in the European Credit Transfer System. Facing the Challenge.
251 pages. 2009. ISBN 978-3-03911-654-6

Vol. 76 Marina Dossena & Ingrid Tieken-Boon van Ostade (eds)
Studies in Late Modern English Correspondence. Methodology and Data.
291 pages. 2008. ISBN 978-3-03911-658-4

Vol. 77 Ingrid Tieken-Boon van Ostade & Wim van der Wurff (eds)
Current Issues in Late Modern English.
436 pages. 2009. ISBN 978-3-03911-660-7

Vol. 78 Marta Navarro Coy (ed.)
Practical Approaches to Foreign Language Teaching and Learning.
297 pages. 2009. ISBN 978-3-03911-661-4

Vol. 79 Qing Ma
Second Language Vocabulary Acquisition.
333 pages. 2009. ISBN 978-3-03911-666-9

Vol. 80 Martin Solly, Michelangelo Conoscenti & Sandra Campagna (eds)
Verbal/Visual Narrative Texts in Higher Education.
384 pages. 2008. ISBN 978-3-03911-672-0

Vol. 81 Meiko Matsumoto
From Simple Verbs to Periphrastic Expressions: The Historical Development of Composite Predicates, Phrasal Verbs, and Related Constructions in English.
235 pages. 2008. ISBN 978-3-03911-675-1

Vol. 82 Melinda Dooly
Doing Diversity. Teachers' Construction of Their Classroom Reality.
180 pages. 2009. ISBN 978-3-03911-687-4

Vol. 83 Victoria Guillén-Nieto, Carmen Marimón-Llorca & Chelo Vargas-Sierra (eds)
Intercultural Business Communication and Simulation and Gaming Methodology.
392 pages. 2009. ISBN 978-3-03911-688-1

Vol. 84 Maria Grazia Guido
English as a Lingua Franca in Cross-cultural Immigration Domains.
285 pages. 2008. ISBN 978-3-03911-689-8

Vol. 85 Erik Castello
Text Complexity and Reading Comprehension Tests.
352 pages. 2008. ISBN 978-3-03911-717-8

Vol. 86 Maria-Lluisa Gea-Valor, Isabel García-Izquierdo & Maria-José Esteve (eds)
Linguistic and Translation Studies in Scientific Communication.
317 pages. 2010. ISBN 978-3-0343-0069-8

Vol. 87 Carmen Navarro, Rosa Mª Rodríguez Abella, Francesca Dalle Pezze & Renzo Miotti (eds)
La comunicación especializada.
355 pages. 2008. ISBN 978-3-03911-733-8

Vol. 88 Kiriko Sato
The Development from Case-Forms to Prepositional Constructions in Old English Prose.
231 pages. 2009. ISBN 978-3-03911-763-5

Vol. 89 Dorothee Heller (Hrsg.)
Formulierungsmuster in deutscher und italienischer Fachkommunikation. Intra- und interlinguale Perspektiven.
315 pages. 2008. ISBN 978-3-03911-778-9

Vol. 90 Henning Bergenholtz, Sandro Nielsen & Sven Tarp (eds)
Lexicography at a Crossroads. Dictionaries and Encyclopedias Today, Lexicographical Tools Tomorrow.
372 pages. 2009. ISBN 978-3-03911-799-4

Vol. 91 Manouchehr Moshtagh Khorasani
The Development of Controversies. From the Early Modern Period to Online Discussion Forums.
317 pages. 2009. ISBN 978-3-3911-711-6

Vol. 92 María Luisa Carrió-Pastor (ed.)
Content and Language Integrated Learning. Cultural Diversity.
178 pages. 2009. ISBN 978-3-3911-818-2

Vol. 93 Roger Berry
Terminology in English Language Teaching. Nature and Use.
262 pages. 2010. ISBN 978-3-0343-0013-1

Vol. 94 Roberto Cagliero & Jennifer Jenkins (eds)
Discourses, Communities, and Global Englishes
240 pages. 2010. ISBN 978-3-0343-0012-4

Vol. 95 Facchinetti Roberta, Crystal David, Seidlhofer Barbara (eds)
From International to Local English – And Back Again.
268 pages. 2010. ISBN 978-3-0343-0011-7

Vol. 96 Cesare Gagliardi & Alan Maley (eds)
EIL, ELF, Global English. Teaching and Learning Issues
376 pages. 2010. ISBN 978-3-0343-0010-0

Vol. 97 Sylvie Hancil (ed.)
The Role of Prosody in Affective Speech.
403 pages. 2009. ISBN 978-3-03911-696-6

Vol. 98 Marina Dossena & Roger Lass (eds)
Studies in English and European Historical Dialectology.
257 pages. 2009. ISBN 978-3-0343-0024-7

Vol. 99 Christine Béal
Les interactions quotidiennes en français et en anglais. De l'approche comparative à l'analyse des situations interculturelles.
424 pages. 2010. ISBN 978-3-0343-0027-8

Vol. 100 Maurizio Gotti (ed.)
Commonality and Individuality in Academic Discourse.
398 pages. 2009. ISBN 978-3-0343-0023-0

Vol. 101 Javier E. Díaz Vera & Rosario Caballero (eds)
Textual Healing. Studies in Medieval English Medical, Scientific and Technical Texts.
213 pages. 2009. ISBN 978-3-03911-822-9

Vol. 102 Nuria Edo Marzá
The Specialised Lexicographical Approach. A Step further in Dictionary-making.
316 pages. 2009. ISBN 978-3-0343-0043-8

Vol. 103 Carlos Prado-Alonso, Lidia Gómez-García, Iria Pastor-Gómez & David Tizón-Couto (eds)
New Trends and Methodologies in Applied English Language Research. Diachronic, Diatopic and Contrastive Studies.
348 pages. 2009. ISBN 978-3-0343-0046-9

Vol. 104 Françoise Salager-Meyer & Beverly A. Lewin
Crossed Words. Criticism in Scholarly Writing?
371 pages. 2011. ISBN 978-3-0343-0049-0.

Vol. 105 Javier Ruano-García
Early Modern Northern English Lexis. A Literary Corpus-Based Study.
611 pages. 2010. ISBN 978-3-0343-0058-2

Vol. 106 Rafael Monroy-Casas
Systems for the Phonetic Transcription of English. Theory and Texts.
280 pages. 2011. ISBN 978-3-0343-0059-9

Vol. 107 Nicola T. Owtram
The Pragmatics of Academic Writing. A Relevance Approach to the Analysis of Research Article Introductions.
311 pages. 2009. ISBN 978-3-0343-0060-5

Vol. 108 Yolanda Ruiz de Zarobe, Juan Manuel Sierra & Francisco Gallardo del Puerto (eds)
Content and Foreign Language Integrated Learning. Contributions to Multilingualism in European Contexts
343 pages. 2011. ISBN 978-3-0343-0074-2

Vol. 109 Ángeles Linde López & Rosalía Crespo Jiménez (eds)
Professional English in the European context. The EHEA challenge.
374 pages. 2010. ISBN 978-3-0343-0088-9

Vol. 110 Rosalía Rodríguez-Vázquez
The Rhythm of Speech, Verse and Vocal Music. A New Theory.
394 pages. 2010. ISBN 978-3-0343-0309-5

Vol. 111 Anastasios Tsangalidis & Roberta Facchinetti (eds)
Studies on English Modality. In Honour of Frank Palmer.
392 pages. 2009. ISBN 978-3-0343-0310-1

Vol. 112 Jing Huang
Autonomy, Agency and Identity in Foreign Language Learning and Teaching.
400 pages. 2013. ISBN 978-3-0343-0370-5

Vol. 113 Mihhail Lotman & Maria-Kristiina Lotman (eds)
Frontiers in Comparative Prosody. In memoriam: Mikhail Gasparov.
426 pages. 2011. ISBN 978-3-0343-0373-6

Vol. 114 Merja Kytö, John Scahill & Harumi Tanabe (eds)
Language Change and Variation from Old English to Late Modern English. A Festschrift for Minoji Akimoto
422 pages. 2010. ISBN 978-3-0343-0372-9

Vol. 115 Giuliana Garzone & Paola Catenaccio (eds)
Identities across Media and Modes. Discursive Perspectives.
379 pages. 2009. ISBN 978-3-0343-0386-6

Vol. 116 Elena Landone
Los marcadores del discurso y cortesía verbal en español.
390 pages. 2010. ISBN 978-3-0343-0413-9

Vol. 117 Maurizio Gotti & Christopher Williams (eds)
Legal Discourse across Languages and Cultures.
339 pages. 2010. ISBN 978-3-0343-0425-2

Vol. 118 David Hirsh
Academic Vocabulary in Context.
217 pages. 2010. ISBN 978-3-0343-0426-9

Vol. 119 Yvonne Dröschel
Lingua Franca English. The Role of Simplification and Transfer.
358 pages. 2011. ISBN 978-3-0343-0432-0

Vol. 120 Tengku Sepora Tengku Mahadi, Helia Vaezian & Mahmoud Akbari
Corpora in Translation. A Practical Guide.
135 pages. 2010. ISBN 978-3-0343-0434-4

Vol. 121 Davide Simone Giannoni & Celina Frade (eds)
Researching Language and the Law. Textual Features and Translation Issues.
278 pages. 2010. ISBN 978-3-0343-0443-6

Vol. 122 Daniel Madrid & Stephen Hughes (eds)
Studies in Bilingual Education.
472 pages. 2011. ISBN 978-3-0343-0474-0

Vol. 123 Vijay K. Bhatia, Christopher N. Candlin & Maurizio Gotti (eds)
The Discourses of Dispute Resolution.
290 pages. 2010. ISBN 978-3-0343-0476-4

Vol. 124 Davide Simone Giannoni
Mapping Academic Values in the Disciplines. A Corpus-Based Approach.
288 pages. 2010. ISBN 978-3-0343-0488-7

Vol. 125 Giuliana Garzone & James Archibald (eds)
Discourse, Identities and Roles in Specialized Communication.
419 pages. 2010. ISBN 978-3-0343-0494-8

Vol. 126 Iria Pastor-Gómez
The Status and Development of N+N Sequences in
Contemporary English Noun Phrases.
216 pages. 2011. ISBN 978-3-0343-0534-1

Vol. 127 Carlos Prado-Alonso
Full-verb Inversion in Written and Spoken English.
261 pages. 2011. ISBN 978-3-0343-0535-8

Vol. 128 Tony Harris & María Moreno Jaén (eds)
Corpus Linguistics in Language Teaching.
214 pages. 2010. ISBN 978-3-0343-0524-2

Vol. 129 Tetsuji Oda & Hiroyuki Eto (eds)
Multiple Perspectives on English Philology and History of Linguistics.
A Festschrift for Shoichi Watanabe on his 80th Birthday.
378 pages. 2010. ISBN 978-3-0343-0480-1

Vol. 130 Luisa Chierichetti & Giovanni Garofalo (eds)
Lengua y Derecho. líneas de investigación interdisciplinaria.
283 pages. 2010. 978-3-0343-0463-4

Vol. 131 Paola Evangelisti Allori & Giuliana Garzone (eds)
Discourse, Identities and Genres in Corporate Communication.
Sponsorship, Advertising and Organizational Communication.
324 pages. 2011. 978-3-0343-0591-4

Vol. 132 Leyre Ruiz de Zarobe & Yolanda Ruiz de Zarobe (eds)
Speech Acts and Politeness across Languages and Cultures.
402 pages. 2012. 978-3-0343-0611-9

Vol. 133 Thomas Christiansen
Cohesion. A Discourse Perspective.
387 pages. 2011. 978-3-0343-0619-5

Vol. 134 Giuliana Garzone & Maurizio Gotti
Discourse, Communication and the Enterprise. Genres and Trends.
451 pages. 2011. ISBN 978-3-0343-0620-1

Vol. 135 Zsuzsa Hoffmann
Ways of the World's Words.
Language Contact in the Age of Globalization.
334 pages 2011. ISBN 978-3-0343-0673-7

Vol. 136 Cecilia Varcasia (ed.)
Becoming Multilingual.
Language Learning and Language Policy between Attitudes and Identities.
213 pages. 2011. ISBN 978-3-0343-0687-5

Vol. 137 Susy Macqueen
The Emergence of Patterns in Second Language Writing.
A Sociocognitive Exploration of Lexical Trails.
325 pages. 2012. ISBN 978-3-0343-1010-9

Vol. 138 Maria Vittoria Calvi & Giovanna Mapelli (eds)
La lengua del turismo. Géneros discursivos y terminología.
365 pages. 2011. ISBN 978-3-0343-1011-6

Vol. 139 Ken Lau
Learning to Become a Professional in a Textually-Mediated World.
A Text-Oriented Study of Placement Practices.
261 pages. 2012. ISBN 978-3-0343-1016-1

Vol. 140 Sandra Campagna, Giuliana Garzone, Cornelia Ilie & Elizabeth Rowley-Jolivet (eds)
Evolving Genres in Web-mediated Communication.
337 pages. 2012. ISBN 978-3-0343-1013-0

Vol. 141 Edith Esch & Martin Solly (eds)
The Sociolinguistics of Language Education in International Contexts.
263 pages. 2012. ISBN 978-3-0343-1009-3

Vol. 142 Forthcoming.

Vol. 143 David Tizón-Couto
Left Dislocation in English. A Functional-Discoursal Approach.
416 pages. 2012. ISBN 978-3-0343-1037-6

Vol. 144 Margrethe Petersen & Jan Engberg (eds)
Current Trends in LSP Research. Aims and Methods.
323 pages. 2011. ISBN 978-3-0343-1054-3

Vol. 145 David Tizón-Couto, Beatriz Tizón-Couto, Iria Pastor-Gómez & Paula Rodríguez-Puente (eds)
New Trends and Methodologies in Applied English Language Research II.
Studies in Language Variation, Meaning and Learning.
283 pages. 2012. ISBN 978-3-0343-1061-1

Vol. 146 Rita Salvi & Hiromasa Tanaka (eds)
Intercultural Interactions in Business and Management.
306 pages. 2011. ISBN 978-3-0343-1039-0

Vol. 147 Francesco Straniero Sergio & Caterina Falbo (eds)
Breaking Ground in Corpus-based Interpreting Studies.
254 pages. 2012. ISBN 978-3-0343-1071-0

Vol. 148 Forthcoming.

Vol. 149 Vijay K. Bhatia & Paola Evangelisti Allori (eds)
Discourse and Identity in the Professions. Legal, Corporate and Institutional Citizenship.
352 pages. 2011. ISBN 978-3-0343-1079-6

Vol. 150 Maurizio Gotti (ed.)
Academic Identity Traits. A Corpus-Based Investigation.
363 pages. 2012. ISBN 978-3-0343-1141-0

Vol. 151 Priscilla Heynderickx, Sylvain Dieltjens, Geert Jacobs, Paul Gillaerts & Elizabeth de Groot (eds)
The Language Factor in International Business.
New Perspectives on Research, Teaching and Practice.
320 pages. 2012. ISBN 978-3-0343-1090-1

Vol. 152 Paul Gillaerts, Elizabeth de Groot, Sylvain Dieltjens, Priscilla Heynderickx & Geert Jacobs (eds)
Researching Discourse in Business Genres. Cases and Corpora.
215 pages. 2012. ISBN 978-3-0343-1092-5

Vol. 153 Yongyan Zheng
Dynamic Vocabulary Development in a Foreign Language.
262 pages. 2012. ISBN 978-3-0343-1106-9

Vol. 154 Carmen Argondizzo (ed.)
Creativity and Innovation in Language Education.
357 pages. 2012. ISBN 978-3-0343-1080-2

Vol. 155 David Hirsh (ed.)
Current Perspectives in Second Language Vocabulary Research.
180 pages. 2012. ISBN 978-3-0343-1108-3

Vol. 156 Seiji Shinkawa
Unhistorical Gender Assignment in Laȝamon's *Brut*. A Case Study of a Late Stage in the Development of Grammatical Gender toward its Ultimate Loss.
186 pages. 2012. ISBN 978-3-0343-1124-3

Vol. 157 Yeonkwon Jung
Basics of Organizational Writing: A Critical Reading Approach.
151 pages. 2014. ISBN 978-3-0343-1137-3.

Vol. 158 Bárbara Eizaga Rebollar (ed.)
Studies in Linguistics and Cognition.
301 pages. 2012. ISBN 978-3-0343-1138-0

Vol. 159 Giuliana Garzone, Paola Catenaccio, Chiara Degano (eds)
Genre Change in the Contemporary World. Short-term Diachronic Perspectives.
329 pages. 2012. ISBN 978-3-0343-1214-1

Vol. 160 Carol Berkenkotter, Vijay K. Bhatia & Maurizio Gotti (eds)
Insights into Academic Genres.
468 pages. 2012. ISBN 978-3-0343-1211-0

Vol. 161 Beatriz Tizón-Couto
Clausal Complements in Native and Learner Spoken English. A corpus-based study with Lindsei and Vicolse. 357 pages. 2013. ISBN 978-3-0343-1184-7

Vol. 162 Patrizia Anesa
Jury Trials and the Popularization of Legal Language. A Discourse Analytical Approach.
247 pages. 2012. ISBN 978-3-0343-1231-8

Vol. 163 David Hirsh
Endangered Languages, Knowledge Systems and Belief Systems.
153 pages. 2013. ISBN 978-3-0343-1232-5

Vol. 164 Eugenia Sainz (ed.)
De la estructura de la frase al tejido del discurso. Estudios contrastivos español/italiano.
305 pages. 2014. ISBN 978-3-0343-1253-0

Vol. 165 Julia Bamford, Franca Poppi & Davide Mazzi (eds)
Space, Place and the Discursive Construction of Identity.
367 pages. 2014. ISBN 978-3-0343-1249-3

Vol. 166 Rita Salvi & Janet Bowker (eds)
Space, Time and the Construction of Identity.
Discursive Indexicality in Cultural, Institutional and Professional Fields.
324 pages. 2013. ISBN 978-3-0343-1254-7

Vol. 167 Shunji Yamazaki & Robert Sigley (eds)
Approaching Language Variation through Corpora. A Festschrift in Honour of Toshio Saito.
421 pages. 2013. ISBN 978-3-0343-1264-6

Vol. 168 Franca Poppi
Global Interactions in English as a Lingua Franca. How written communication is changing under the influence of electronic media and new contexts of use.
249 pages. 2012. ISBN 978-3-0343-1276-9

Vol. 169 Miguel A. Aijón Oliva & María José Serrano
Style in syntax. Investigating variation in Spanish pronoun subjects.
239 pages. 2013. ISBN 978-3-0343-1244 8

Vol. 170 Inés Olza, Óscar Loureda & Manuel Casado-Velarde (eds)
Language Use in the Public Sphere. Methodological Perspectives and Empirical Applications
564 pages. 2014. ISBN 978-3-0343-1286-8

Vol. 171 Aleksandra Matulewska
Legilinguistic Translatology. A Parametric Approach to Legal Translation.
279 pages. 2013. ISBN 978-3-0343-1287-5

Vol. 172 Maurizio Gotti & Carmen Sancho Guinda (eds)
Narratives in Academic and Professional Genres.
513 pages. 2013. ISBN 978-3-0343-1371-1

Vol. 173 Madalina Chitez
Learner corpus profiles. The case of Romanian Learner English.
244 pages. 2014. ISBN 978-3-0343-1410-7

Vol. 174 Chihiro Inoue
Task Equivalence in Speaking Tests.
251 pages. 2013. ISBN 978-3-0343-1417-6

Vol. 175 Gabriel Quiroz & Pedro Patiño (eds.)
LSP in Colombia: advances and challenges.
339 pages. 2014. ISBN 978-3-0343-1434-3

Vol. 176 Catherine Resche
Economic Terms and Beyond: Capitalising on the Wealth of Notions.
How Researchers in Specialised Varieties of English Can Benefit from Focusing on Terms.
332 pages. 2013. ISBN 978-3-0343-1435-0

Vol. 177 Forthcoming.

Vol. 178 Cécile Desoutter & Caroline Mellet (dir.)
Le discours rapporté: approches linguistiques et perspectives didactiques.
270 pages. 2013. ISBN 978-3-0343-1292-9

Vol. 179 Ana Díaz-Negrillo & Francisco Javier Díaz-Pérez (eds)
Specialisation and Variation in Language Corpora.
341 pages. 2014. ISBN 978-3-0343-1316-2

Vol. 180 Pilar Alonso
A Multi-dimensional Approach to Discourse Coherence. From Standardness to Creativity.
247 pages. 2014. ISBN 978-3-0343-1325-4

Vol. 181 Alejandro Alcaraz-Sintes & Salvador Valera-Hernández (eds)
Diachrony and Synchrony in English Corpus Linguistics.
393 pages. 2014. ISBN 978-3-0343-1326-1

Vol. 182 Runhan Zhang
Investigating Linguistic Knowledge of a Second Language.
207 pages. 2015. ISBN 978-3-0343-1330-8

Vol. 183 Hajar Abdul Rahim & Shakila Abdul Manan (eds.)
English in Malaysia. Postcolonial and Beyond.
267 pages. 2014. ISBN 978-3-0343-1341-4

Vol. 184 Virginie Fasel Lauzon
Comprendre et apprendre dans l'interaction. Les séquences d'explication en classe de français langue seconde.
292 pages. 2014. ISBN 978-3-0343-1451-0

Vol. 185 Forthcoming.

Vol. 186 Wei Ren
L2 Pragmatic Development in Study Abroad Contexts
256 pages. 2015. ISBN 978-3-0343-1358-2

Vol. 187 Marina Bondi & Rosa Lorés Sanz (eds)
Abstracts in Academic Discourse. Variation and Change.
361 pages. 2014. ISBN 978-3-0343-1483-1

Vol. 188 Forthcoming.

Vol. 189 Paola Evangelisti Allori (ed.)
Identities in and across Cultures.
315 pages. 2014. ISBN 978-3-0343-1458-9

Vol. 190 Erik Castello, Katherine Ackerley & Francesca Coccetta (eds).
Studies in Learner Corpus Linguistics. Research and Applications for Foreign Language Teaching and Assessment.
358 pages. 2015. ISBN 978-3-0343-1506-7

Vol. 191 Ruth Breeze, Maurizio Gotti & Carmen Sancho Guinda (eds)
Interpersonality in Legal Genres.
389 pages. 2014. ISBN 978-3-0343-1524-1

Vol. 192 Paola Evangelisti Allori, John Bateman & Vijay K. Bhatia (eds)
Evolution in Genre. Emergence, Variation, Multimodality.
364 pages. 2014. ISBN 978-3-0343-1533-3

Vol. 193 Jiyeon Kook
Agency in Arzt-Patient-Gesprächen. Zur interaktionistischen Konzeptualisierung von Agency
271 pages. 2015. ISBN 978-3-0343-1666-8

Vol. 194 Susana Nicolás Román & Juan José Torres Núñez (eds)
Drama and CLIL. A new challenge for the teaching approaches in bilingual education.
170 pages. 2015. ISBN 978-3-0343-1629-3

Vol. 195 Alessandra Molino & Serenella Zanotti (eds)
Observing Norm, Observing Usage. Lexis in Dictionaries and in the Media.
430 pages. 2015. ISBN 978-3-0343-1584-5

Vol. 196 Begoña Soneira
A Lexical Description of English for Architecture. A Corpus-based Approach.
267 pages. 2015. ISBN 978-3-0343-1602-6

Vol. 197 M Luisa Roca-Varela
False Friends in Learner Corpora. A corpus-based study of English false friends in the written and spoken production of Spanish learners.
348 pages. 2015. ISBN 978-3-0343-1620-0

Vol. 198 Rahma Al-Mahrooqi & Christopher Denman
Bridging the Gap between Education and Employment. English Language Instruction in EFL Contexts.
416 pages. 2015. ISBN 978-3-0343-1681-1

Vol. 199 Rita Salvi & Janet Bowker (eds)
The Dissemination of Contemporary Knowledge in English. Genres, discourse strategies and professional practices.
171 pages. 2015. ISBN 978-3-0343-1679-8

Vol. 200 Maurizio Gotti & Davide S. Giannoni (eds)
Corpus Analysis for Descriptive and Pedagogical Purposes. ESP Perspectives.
432 pages. 2014. ISBN 978-3-0343-1516-6

Vol. 201 Ida Ruffolo
The Perception of Nature in Travel Promotion Texts. A Corpus-based Discourse Analysis.
148 pages. 2015. ISBN 978-3-0343-1521-0

Vol. 202 Ives Trevian
English suffixes. Stress-assignment properties, productivity, selection and combinatorial processes.
471 pages. 2015. ISBN 978-3-0343-1576-0

Vol. 203 Maurizio Gotti, Stefania Maci & Michele Sala (eds)
Insights into Medical Communication.
422 pages. 2015. ISBN 978-3-0343-1694-1

Vol. 204 Carmen Argondizzo (ed.)
European Projects in University Language Centres. Creativity, Dynamics, Best Practice.
371 pages. 2015. ISBN 978-3-0343-1696-5

Vol. 205 Aura Luz Duffé Montalván (ed.)
Estudios sobre el léxico. Puntos y contrapuntos.
502 pages. 2016. ISBN 978-3-0343-2011-5

Vol. 206 Maria Pavesi, Maicol Formentelli & Elisa Ghia (eds)
The Languages of Dubbing. Mainstream Audiovisual Translation in Italy.
275 pages. 2014. ISBN 978-3-0343-1646-0

Vol. 207 Forthcoming.

Vol. 208 Vijay K. Bhatia & Maurizio Gotti (eds)
Arbitration Discourse in Asia.
331 pages. 2015. ISBN 978-3-0343-2032-0

Vol. 209 Forthcoming.

Vol. 210 Francisco Alonso Almeida, Laura Cruz García & Víctor González Ruiz (eds)
Corpus-based studies on language varieties.
285 pages. 2016. ISBN 978-3-0343-2044-3

Vol. 211 Juan Pedro Rica Peromingo
Aspectos lingüísticos y técnicos de la traducción audiovisual (TAV).
177 pages. 2016. ISBN 978-3-0343-2055-9

Vol. 212 Forthcoming.

Vol. 213 Zhilong Xie
Bilingual Advantages. Contributions of Different Bilingual Experiences to Cognitive Control Differences Among Young-adult Bilinguals.
238 pages. 2016. ISBN 978-3-0343-2081-8

Vol. 214 Larissa D'Angelo
Academic posters. A textual and visual metadiscourse analysis.
367 pages. 2016. ISBN 978-3-0343-2083-2

Vol. 215 Evelyne Berger
Prendre la parole en L2. Regard sur la compétence d'interaction en classe de langue.
246 pages. 2016. ISBN 978-3-0343-2084-9

Vol. 216 David Lasagabaster and Aintzane Doiz (eds)
CLIL experiences in secondary and tertiary education: In search of good practices.
262 pages. 2016. ISBN 978-3-0343-2104-4

Vol. 217 Forthcoming.

Vol. 218 Sandra Campagna, Elana Ochse, Virginia Pulcini & Martin Solly (eds)
Languaging in and across Communities: New Voices, New Identities. Studies in Honour of Giuseppina Cortese.
507 pages. 2016. ISBN 978-3-0343-2073-3

Vol. 219 Adriana Orlandi & Laura Giacomini (ed.)
Defining collocation for lexicographic purposes. From linguistic theory to lexicographic practice.
328 pages. 2016. ISBN 978-3-0343-2054-2

www.ingramcontent.com/pod-product-compliance
Ingram Content Group UK Ltd.
Pitfield, Milton Keynes, MK11 3LW, UK
UKHW020200290926
15471UKWH00005B/978

9 783034 320818